TAI CHI

PAUL CROMPTON has studied Tai Chi and other martial arts for over 40 years, and is an internationally recognized expert in these arts. He began teaching Tai Chi in 1968 in London, and then went to work with several different teachers over the next 30 years, as well as teaching to others. As well as teaching Tai Chi, he has also studied meditation, Chi Kung and various other subjects such as Judo, Karate, Aikido and various branches of Kung Fu. Though interested in martial arts, he has always looked to them for the therapeutic, internal aspects that these subjects can provide. He has written extensively on the martial arts, and his books include *A Practical Introduction: Tai Chi and Walking Meditation.*

THE SERIES

New Perspectives provide attractive and accessible introductions to a comprehensive range of mind, body and spirit topics. Beautifully designed and illustrated, these practical books are written by experts in each subject.

Titles in the series include:

ASTROLOGY
by Janis Huntley

I CHING
by Stephen Karcher

BUDDHISM
by John Snelling

NUTRITIONAL THERAPY
by Jeannette Ewin

CHAKRAS
by Naomi Ozaniec

RUNES
by Bernard King

COLOUR THERAPY
by Pauline Wills

SHAMANISM
by Nevill Drury

CRYSTAL THERAPY
by Stephanie Harrison & Tim Harrison

TAI CHI
by Paul Crompton

HERBAL REMEDIES
by Vicki Pitman

YOGA
by Howard Kent

New Perspectives

TAI CHI

An Introductory Guide to the Chinese Art of Movement

PAUL CROMPTON

ELEMENT

Shaftesbury, Dorset • Boston, Massachusetts
Melbourne, Victoria

First published as *The Elements of Tai Chi*
in 1990 by Element Books Limited

This revised edition first published in Great Britain in 2000 by
Element Books Limited, Shaftesbury, Dorset SP7 8BP

Published in the USA in 2000 by Element Books, Inc.
160 North Washington Street,
Boston, MA 02114

Published in Australia in 2000 by
Element Books and distributed by
Penguin Australia Limited,
487 Maroondah Highway, Ringwood,
Victoria 3134

Designed for Element Books Limited by
Design Revolution, Queens Park Villa,
30 West Drive, Brighton, East Sussex BN2 2GE

ELEMENT BOOKS LIMITED
Editorial Director: Sarah Sutton
Project Editor: Kelly Wakely
Commissioning Editor: Grace Cheetham
Production Director: Roger Lane

DESIGN REVOLUTION
Editorial Director: Ian Whitelaw
Art Director: Lindsey Johns
Project Editor: Nicola Hodgson
Editor: Julie Whitaker
Designer: Lucie Penn

Printed and bound in Great Britain by
Bemrose Security Printing, Derby

British Library Cataloguing in Publication
Data available

Library of Congress Cataloging in Publication
Data available

ISBN 1-86204-760-X

CONTENTS

Author's Note

This new edition of the book *Elements of Tai Chi*, newly designed and set, will appeal to all those who are interested in Tai Chi. The first edition was welcomed both by my peers and those less well informed about the art. It was even included in the reading list of an English university course in comparative religious studies. The publishers have chosen to illustrate this edition with photographs, which they thought would be in keeping with the new design.

Acknowledgements

The publishers wish to thank The Bridgeman Art Library for the use of the picture on page 10.

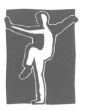

INTRODUCTION

Moving slowly, under the trees, breathing, it seems, in time with a gentle breeze; merging with Nature itself in a healing rhythm. Head, shoulders, arms, trunk, legs and feet moving as one; continuously, smoothly and restfully; as if swimming into a new, all-pervading element; a different time, a different space.

Poor words, but an attempt to convey the experience of performing the movements of T'ai Chi Ch'uan, the Chinese art of soft and gentle exercise. Western usage has reduced the full expression to Tai Chi, and this abbreviation will be used throughout this book.

Tai Chi is said to be the child of Taoist teachings, but its historical origins have disappeared into the mists of the past. Nonetheless, the history of Taoism itself throws some light on the history of Tai Chi, for they both demonstrate two levels of understanding. The earliest and deeper level of Taoism taught a way of understanding the relationship between humans and the universe by indicating that any attempt by humans to 'do' or to interfere with the natural order of things was an error, based on ignorance of the workings of the Tao. The Tao (pronounced 'Dow'), the Way of Heaven, was displayed in the natural order of things, and humans could only perceive this natural order by becoming one with it; not by analysis and manipulation. The later, degenerated form of Taoist religion became mixed with magic, occultism, manipulation of energy and interference with the natural order.

Contaminated by other influences, foreign to its nature, Tai Chi today is little more than a reminder that at one time the people who studied and practised it had real knowledge of the place of humans in the universe. Throughout Chinese history, eminent and obscure Taoists influenced behaviour and thought at many levels of society. Their influence was felt by scholars, farmers, Mongolian khans and emperors. But that time has gone, the source has gone, and now we have a situation in which here and there in different parts of the world there are some respected Taoists and Tai Chi masters, but the entire context into which Taoism was born and flourished, and into which the art of Tai Chi was introduced, no longer exists.

Professor Fung Yu-lan, author of *A Short History of Chinese Philosophy*, points out that Chinese philosophy is expressed in the form of 'suggestive', pithy maxims. Their brevity is meant to inspire 'reflective thinking', and contrasts with the 'articulate' pronouncements of Western philosophy, which aim to be as exact and explicit as possible. This contrast between suggestion and articulate expression has spread into the study and teaching of Tai Chi in a manner that causes confusion. We find in the writings of some Tai Chi teachers, especially modern ones, a mixture of fact, misinformation, wisdom, fantasy and poetic imagery.

The suggestive aphorisms of the Taoist philosophy are meant to evoke a mood in which the movements of Tai Chi are performed. Through Western influences there has been an influx of attempted *articulate suggestions* – a contradiction in terms. There can be no articulate explanation of the necessary mood. The best known book of Taoist wisdom is the *Tao Te Ching*. The opening lines read:

> *'The Tao that is expressed in words*
> *is not the true Tao.'*

The whole book creates a mood, an attitude towards life, and the wise sayings that are used in Tai Chi books should be approached in the same way. They are like many sticks of incense of different flavours all burning simultaneously to produce an overall scent. This scent should inform the Tai Chi movements.

So different threads run through this book, producing, it is hoped, a tapestry of Tai Chi such as any student of the art might weave, for himself or herself. For us Westerners, this is preferable to trying to adopt either the suggestive or articulate approach exclusively, because to do so would be artificial. We need to find our own understanding of Tai Chi.

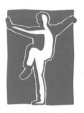

THE HISTORY
OF TAI CHI

CHAPTER ONE

Chinese people have emigrated and settled in just about every country in the world. This has meant that Chinese culture has taken root everywhere, and this culture includes the art of Tai Chi. Consequently, any history of Tai Chi would have to be encyclopaedic if it were to be comprehensive.

CHANG SAN-FENG

All accounts of the history of Tai Chi make mention of the legendary Chang San-feng. He was a Taoist Immortal; eccentric, playful, over two metres tall, a formidable fighter, always unkempt in appearance and immensely strong.

Being an immortal, he could have existed at any time, and the many accounts of his life and references to him bear this out. A hundred years before the Ming dynasty, in the 13th century, he is written about as the friend of a well-known figure, Liu Ping-chung (1216–1274), a

LEFT THREE OF THE EARLY FOUNDERS OF TAOISM. TAI CHI IS BASED ON THIS ANCIENT CHINESE PHILOSOPHY.

Ch'an monk connected with Kubilai Khan. In the Sung dynasty (960–1279), Chang San-feng appears from time to time. From 1368 to 1398 he is supposed to have travelled in Szechwan. During his travels, he stayed with a certain family and used to sit in meditation in their garden. One day, he planted some branches of a plum tree in the ground as he sat and they immediately burst into blossom. Later still he was glimpsed in Shantung province riding on the back of a flying crane. In 1459 he was made a saint by Emperor Ying-tsun. The name of Immortal Penetrating Mystery and Revealing Transformation was conferred upon him. One of the places he stayed in, the Wu-tang peak district in northern Hopei, was to become famous in Tai Chi history. It was already an abode of Taoist hermits and home of the god of war, Hsuan-lang, who had a shrine built there in his honour.

The earliest known mention of Chang San-feng as a martial artist is found in the biography of a well known boxing master of the time, Chang Sung-ch'i, who lived in the 16th century, in Ning-po. Chang Sung-ch'i said that he had been taught his art by an alchemist called Chang San-feng who lived as a hermit on the Wu-tang peaks. The name given to the fighting methods that Chang Sung-ch'i used is not Tai Chi, as one might expect, but 'Nei-chia' or 'internal/esoteric school'. Some writers have maintained that Nei Chia and Tai Chi are the same, but the more impartial writers point out that this is a mistake. Part of the evidence for refuting this link comes from a stone epitaph for a certain Wang Cheng-nan, who lived in the 17th century. The epitaph shows that Chang passed on his methods of fighting from teacher to teacher until it reached Wang Cheng-nan himself. Wang Cheng-nan's style of boxing was called Nei Chia. So, if Chang San-feng lived at all, he was probably connected to Nei Chia alone.

HSU HSUN-PING

A second theory about the origins of Tai Chi is that it began during the T'ang dynasty (618–907). It is said that there were four separate schools of martial arts. The founder of the first was a hermit called Hsu Hsun-ping (Hsa Suan-ming). His style was called the Three

Generations and Seven, and it consisted of 37 postures containing the Eight Trigrams in the arm movements and the Five Elements in the leg movements (*see* chapter 7). It was said that his style was based on the understanding of the I-Ching.

The founder of the second school, called Long Ch'uan or Long Fist/Boxing, was Li Tao-tzu, another Immortal. Of the other two schools there is little to say, except that they were created by Yin Li-hsiang and Cheng Ling-si. Legend says that Chang San-feng integrated the four schools into one, to make Tai Chi but there is no hard evidence to prove that this was so.

WANG TSUNG-YUEH

A third claim gives the credit for founding Tai Chi to Wang Tsung-yueh of Shansi. One day he was passing through a Chen family village in Honan province sometime between 1736 and 1795. Before going to rest at the village inn for the night, he paused to watch some of the locals training in martial arts. As a traveller he was an object of respectful curiosity and was soon engaged in conversation. He made some passing remark about the standard of martial arts in the village and this provoked a number of challenges from the Chen villagers. Wang accepted them and trounced them all. His method of fighting was 'soft' or internal, not relying solely on strength and force. This impressed the Chen fraternity and the leaders of the village asked Wang to stay on and teach them. He agreed, and this marked the beginning of the Chen style of Tai Chi in China.

CHEN WANG-T'ING

The last account of the origins of Tai Chi is the account most favoured by the Chen family descendants, mainly because it gives the inspiration for creating Tai Chi firmly to the Chen family. According to this theory, the founding of Tai Chi took place during the Ming dynasty (1368–1654). However, the Chen family give credit to other styles of martial arts upon which its founder, Chen Wang-t'ing based his creation.

Chen Wang-t'ing studied many martial arts in his youth; he combined deep breathing and mental concentration with animal movement exercises. He studied the theories of Chinese traditional medicine and invented turning, arcing and spiral movements, which purported to stimulate the Chi energy running along the acupuncture channels. He introduced movements that alternate between the two extremes of yang, hard, and yin, soft. He also invented the two person Push Hands training exercises (*see* p.52). He also developed the use of the Tai Chi spear, in particular the 'sticking spear' methods.

However, not all the new forms of Tai Chi movement invented by Chen Wang-t'ing survived. He passed on seven sets of Tai Chi boxing routines but after only a few generations there were few people who could do the whole syllabus of training. Chen Yu-pun created the New Style, which did away with the more difficult techniques. Chen Ch'ing-p'ing produced a slower style, which was more compact in its movements. There then existed three styles of Chen family Tai Chi – what remained of the Old Style, the New Style of Chen Yu-pun and the Chen style of Chen Ch'ing-p'ing. The remnants of the Old Style were brought to Peking in 1928 by Chen Fake. From then on this branch of the Chen style underwent various changes but still survives and thrives in China today.

CHENG MAN-CH'ING

Cheng Man-ch'ing, sometimes written Cheng Man-jan, deserves a special place in this chapter because of the wide influence his teachings and writings have had in the West.

Cheng was born in Chekiang province in 1901. His father died when he was a small child and Cheng was very much influenced by his mother, who taught him poetry and calligraphy. He also attended school near Mount Kuang-lu, and in his spare time he would visit Buddhist temples in the vicinity. Cheng had an extraordinarily good memory and it is said that by the age of nine he had memorized the classics of Confucian teaching. By the age of 14, he was sufficiently skilled at painting to be able to support his family. The gift for

YANG LU-CH'AN

The famous founder of the Yang family style, Yang Lu-ch'an, is said to have gained access to the closely guarded secrets of the Chen family by spying on them from a hidden vantage point and memorizing what he had seen. After no less than ten years of trying to learn on his own, he was finally discovered by Chen family members who ordered him to show them what he had achieved. Such was his skill and fidelity to the art that he was accepted as a student; a rare step in those days. He learned the Old Style, but gradually changed it and adapted it as a method of keeping fit rather than as a method of fighting. This modified Chen style was learned by the third son of Yang Lu-ch'an, Yang Chien-hou, who taught it under the name of Middle Style. The third son of Yang Chien-hou, Yang Cheng-fu, studied under his father and he changed the movements into a slow, continuous and graceful style that he called the Big Style. The Big Style became the basis of most of the Tai Chi that is practised in the West today. It is best known in two solo forms; the Long Form and the Short Form of Cheng Man-ch'ing.

THE OLD WU STYLE

Wu Yu-seong, who began studying Tai Chi with Yang Lu-ch'an and later went to Chen Ch'ing-p'ing, founded his own Wu style, which later became known as the Old Wu Style.

There are two Wu styles in existence today. One is the Old Style of Wu Yu-seong, initially based on the Yang Lu-ch'an and Chen Ch'ing-p'ing styles. The other originated from Wu Chien-ch'uan, a pupil of Ch'uan Yu who had learned from Yang Lu-ch'an. This second style spread to Singapore and is popular there.

painting was echoed in the fields of medicine, calligraphy, classical studies, poetry and martial arts. Before Cheng took up martial arts, he suffered from rheumatism, beriberi and tuberculosis; the latter reaching a stage where he coughed up blood. He was not expected to survive this illness, which was widespread in China at that time. Then a friend introduced him to Yang Cheng-fu, who was already renowned for his Tai Chi skills. Cheng began to study Tai Chi and his health improved. As soon as it did so, he stopped training and his illness came back. Filled with regret at his folly, Cheng began to train again and his health improved until he became quite robust. From then on he trained daily without fail. In Taiwan he established the Shr Jung School of Tai Chi. He died in Taipei on March 26, 1975.

Cheng's first and eldest student, who became more of a disciple, was T'ung Tsai Liang, born in Hopei province in 1900. Liang was with Cheng for 20 years and became a respected teacher in his own right. He assisted Cheng with work at the United Nations in New York and also taught at Boston College, Harvard University, Amherst and other American colleges.

What characterizes Cheng's handed-down form of Tai Chi training, as far as one can gather, is its softness, its humanity, and the relative smallness of the movements compared with the large movements of Yang Cheng-fu, his teacher, and Chen Wei-ming. A story current for many years among Chinese martial artists is that Cheng changed what he had learned from Yang and produced his Short Form for the sake of Western students whom he initially thought would be unable or unwilling to do the more strenuous Long Form.

MADAM BOW-SIM MARK

A leading and innovative teacher of modern times is Madam Bow-Sim Mark, currently head of the Chinese Wushu Research Institute in Boston, Massachusetts in the US. From childhood she studied the Yang and Wu styles of Tai Chi and later the Combined Form, a modern series of movements that incorporates actions from several styles. Her meticulous attention to detail and her ten hours a day

YANG CHENG-FU

Yang Cheng-fu, (1883–1936), is the most written-about Tai Chi master of the 20th century in Hong Kong and mainland China. As a child he had no liking for the art and only took it up seriously in his early 20s. On the death of his father his whole attitude changed and he began to try to plumb the depths of Tai Chi. He took up residence in Shanghai and taught martial arts there in a special school. During this period, Yang's Tai Chi was said to be very powerful, with fast-kicking techniques. From what we know of the Chen style, it seems as though Yang's art still owed a lot to that style's variations in speed, its power and size of movement.

Then Yang began to realize that Tai Chi could do a lot for the treatment of chronic diseases, building up one's health and promoting long life. He started to introduce modifications into what he had been taught and reorganized the movements of the forms into one long, slow and continuous series, aimed at stimulating the health of students. He relegated fighting to a less prominent role.

16

SUN LU-TANG

Sun Lu-tang (1860–1932) was an example of a man who first studied other martial arts and then came to Tai Chi. He was one of the chief exponents in his time of Hsing-I Ch'uan and Pa-kua Ch'uan, the other two internal martial arts of China. He studied under Hao Wei-chen, a pupil of Li I-yu. In his early years, he had fits of depression and twice attempted suicide. His training in martial arts swept this tendency away and he became a famous fighter, but one who shunned attention. In his later years, he blended his Tai Chi with the other two arts and founded his own recognized style, Sun Style.

training programme marked her out as a future master. She went on to study Pa-kua Ch'uan and various sword forms. Respected and admired both in China and the United States, she has been the promulgating spearhead of the new forms of Tai Chi that have emerged since the early 1950s.

This chapter shows us a number of things that are worth emphasizing. One is that training in Tai Chi is a long and arduous process if a high standard is desired. Secondly, the known history of the art shows that a wide variety of movements, of differing speeds, executed with varying degrees of power are the basis of whatever is taught today. Lastly, the influences of Taoist philosophy and religion need to be much more closely examined before they can be confirmed.

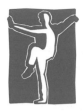

THE POSTURES
AND MOVEMENTS
OF TAI CHI

CHAPTER TWO

The chequered and controversial history of Tai Chi should be borne in mind when reading the remainder of this book, especially in connection with the postures and movements. It is said that the original postures were assumed separately from one another, and that at some unknown point they were joined together into a continuous series of movements that is generally referred to as the 'form'.

A form is found in all Eastern martial arts. Some martial arts have many forms. Within the form we find all the movements and postures characteristic of the art in question. By doing the forms, students are constantly reminded of and trained in the style itself. The postures can be thought of as places on a map that one passes through, and the movements as the roads that connect the postures together. So a form is a kind of moving map. A Tai Chi teacher shows the postures to the class, corrects them and tries to ensure that they are done well. Such are the differences in physical build and temperament that no two people will take a given posture in exactly the same way. But even to an outsider, it will be plain that a posture of a Single Whip for example, is being taken by a class of students, however much they may differ from one another.

Another strongly held belief among Tai Chi adherents is that originally there were 13 postures or movements. In the course of time, with, as we have seen, the influence of different teachers, other postures and intermediate movements were added, and variations in the positions of arms, legs, trunk and head were introduced. This tendency extended so far as to produce different styles of Tai Chi, in which the same names were given to postures that could not reasonably be called the *same*, although certain similarities often remained. An example of this is once again the Single Whip posture, which has several variations, but can only be identified by the singular way in which one hand is held in a beak-like formation with the fingers and thumbs joined at the tips.

Many Tai Chi enthusiasts are very partisan. Their attitude to the art is critical of other styles, and they commonly say that this or that way of doing Tai Chi is wrong. In general, the more cautious students see this attitude as nonsensical, since no one knows what the original postures were like. Photographs of the famous Tai Chi master, Yang Cheng-fu, both as a young and an old man show differences in posture, but these could be attributed to age and change in build. Yang Cheng-fu's own explanation was that his posture was better when he was older.

Like any other subject that is highly specialized, Tai Chi does produce in many of its followers a close attention to detail. To an outsider, the exact position of a foot or hand may seem trivial. To someone who is closely involved in the art, a slight shift of the weight or the turning in or out of the foot some ten degrees makes a big difference, because an aware student experiences these small changes as a definite physical sensation. Such details then play an important part in the smooth performance of the forms, and repeated wrong positions can produce injury to a joint or muscle strain, especially at the knees. Students who have been correctly taught become sensitive to details and once proficient they can usually adapt quickly to another form or style under the guidance of a competent teacher.

POSTURES AND THE EIGHT TRIGRAMS

The most important postures are said by some teachers to be directly related to the Eight Trigrams of the *I-Ching* (see chapter 7). These are:

WARD OFF *(P'eng)*	equated with trigram Chien	*Moving in the*
ROLL-BACK *(Lu)*	equated with trigram Kun	*four major*
PRESS *(Chi)*	equated with trigram Kan	*compass*
PUSH *(An)*	equated with trigram Li	*directions*
PULL *(Tsai)*	equated with trigram Sun	*Moving in the*
SPLIT *(Lieh)*	equated with trigram Chen	*four major*
ELBOW *(Chou)*	equated with trigram Tai	*compass*
SHOULDER *(Kao)*	equated with trigram Ken	*directions*

This makes eight postures, and to these should be added the Five Steps, which are linked by some teachers with the Five Elements (see chapter 7).

ADVANCING	related to the element metal
RETREATING	related to the element wood
LOOKING LEFT	related to the element water
LOOKING RIGHT	related to the element fire
EQUILIBRIUM	related to the element earth

The Eight Postures are sometimes called Gates, Pa-men. Wu Pu is the Chinese for Five Steps.

These 13 movement-postures are the basis for the Yang style of Tai Chi. Although the Eight Gates are theoretically connected with the eight directions of the compass, they do not follow these directions in the forms.

20

THE EIGHT POSTURES OR GATES

1. WARD OFF (P'ENG)

In the Chen style, a movement similar to Ward Off is assumed as one of the current form's beginnings. In it, the feet are spread wide apart as if riding a very large horse.

We find two versions in the Yang style of Yang Cheng-fu. One is exemplified by Cheng Man-ch'ing, with the left hand raised in front of the chest, the right arm lowered in front of and to the side of the thigh and the rear foot turned in about 45 degrees. The other, seen in old photographs, shows Yang himself with the rear foot turned out at 90 degrees to the forward facing direction and the arms in a slightly different position from that of Cheng. Also, the torso is held differently. The Combined Tai Chi form, which is a synthesis produced in 1956 in China, and taught in the West by Bow-Sim Mark, has a similar position to that held by Yang Cheng-fu.

In the version of the Wu style that travelled to Singapore, the opening movements of the form show a Ward Off posture with the trunk inclined well forward, and the hands in a different position from that of the Yang or Chen styles. Because the trigram for P'eng shows three unbroken or strong lines, yang or masculine lines (for examples of the trigrams, *see* p.94), then the movement itself is associated by some teachers with the supreme source of power and strength, the heavens.

It should be explained to Tai Chi beginners who question how Ward Off can be used in self defence or Push Hands, that, in addition to its use with the palm turned in, which can denote either an attacking or defending action, it has a use with the palm

21

LEFT ENTERING INTO WARD OFF. THE WARD OFF POSTURE, WHICH IS EQUATED WITH THE CHIEN TRIGRAM, IS ASSOCIATED WITH THE HEAVENS.

turned out, an attack. Right at the moment when Ward Off is completed, and the hands turn outwards to go into Roll-Back, one can push with both hands at the same time. This is not apparent in learning the form because students are usually preoccupied with the transition from one movement to the other and the significance of the small hand Ward Off, as in all the other postures, relaxation and correct use of change escapes all but the most alert. For the correct performance of Ward Off, as in all the other postures, relaxation and correct use of strength and balance should be observed. Speaking in general, this has to be learned from a teacher. There are few Western students who have what one could call a natural propensity for Tai Chi movement.

2. ROLL-BACK (LU)

The second movement of the Yang form, after left and right Ward Off, is done in a deep crouching stance in the Chen form. In the Yang form, it is taken much higher, with again the two foot variations described for Ward Off. In the Wu style, the trunk is again inclined. As the trigram for Lu consists of three broken or yin lines, this indicates that the posture or movement of Roll-Back is one of yielding, par excellence. It is the antithesis of the offensive, yang of Ward Off. At the same time, in application to self defence, the Roll-Back can include seizing the partner by the arm and pulling, yang, as well as the deflecting or diverting on the forearm, yin.

Within every yang, some yin; within every yin, some yang. This procession of defence, offense, defence or contraction and expansion is said to reflect the natural

LEFT ROLL-BACK, WHICH IS LARGELY A YIELDING MOVEMENT, CAN DEFLECT A STRIKE OR PUSH FROM AN OPPONENT. IT IS ASSOCIATED WITH THE KUN TRIGRAM, MEANING RECEPTIVITY.

world of seasons, waxing and waning of the moon, light and darkness and so on. One would therefore expect the next movement to be mainly yang, and in the form this is so.

3. PRESS (CHI)

In this posture, the yin and yang lines combine for the first time in the trigram with one yin, broken line on top, one yang unbroken line in the middle and a yin line at the bottom. Looked at very simply, this arrangement indicates yang concealed in yin, cocooned in yin. This can be interpreted to mean that in doing Press in Push Hands, the initial contact with the partner is soft, the yin line, to sense his or her balance. If this is known, then the hard, yang line is used so to speak to uproot and throw off balance. Because this bright yang force is shrouded in the mist of yin, the action of Chi, or Press, is sometimes described as the most deceptive and dangerous.

In Chen style, it is carried out in a very low stance with one leg stretched out and the other bent, the waist turning strongly to the right. In Wu style, the performer presses down and then expands forward, inclining the trunk with hands joined. In Yang style, the left hand touches the right forearm or the heel of the hand, in all cases standing upright as a rule but one sometimes sees it with a small inclination forward of the trunk. In the simplified 24 Step Peking form, the fingers of the left hand lightly rest on the pulse of the right wrist. Another variation is to press with palm against palm.

This posture is a suitable one for showing the detail and variations, which were mentioned earlier. When the hands are joined in any of the ways just described, it seems as though the

23

RIGHT PRESS IS DESCRIBED AS A DECEPTIVE MOVEMENT, SINCE THE FORCE OF YANG IS CONCEALED WITHIN THE SOFTNESS OF YIN.

back of the right hand and forearm will be used to uproot and throw away a partner. This is quite feasible and often Press is used in this way. However, this could be seen as a yin phase of the contact where the balance is once more sensed and then, as the hands separate to withdraw, a push could be made with both palms, facing away from the body. A different use of Press can be to use both hands, joined, to make a shock strike at the solar plexus of an opponent with the back of the right hand.

4. PUSH (AN)

In one version of the Wu style Push, it is performed with the right hand leading and the body inclined. In the Chen style, it begins from the deep horse-riding position followed by bringing the feet closer and rising to a standing-up position. In both Chen and Yang styles, the hands push together, though some teachers maintain that the hands should never push equally in force as this is called 'double weighting' of the hands. A similar dictum, 'no double weighting in the feet', is echoed by many teachers. This means that the weight of the body should never be evenly distributed on both feet as this makes one susceptible to being pushed off balance more easily.

In all styles, the mode of pushing is subject to variations. Beginners will generally be taught to push in a straight line, subject to the teacher's preferences, and then a curving push should be introduced, something like the shape of a mounting wave. In this curving push, the hands usually push down towards the waist first and then rise gradually

RIGHT WHEN PERFORMING THE PUSH MOVEMENT, TAKE CARE NOT TO LET THE KNEE EXTEND BEYOND THE TOES AS THIS MAY CAUSE INSTABILITY.

upwards and forwards. If the action of Push is done repeatedly for training purposes, then the hands will complete a kind of horizontal oval shape, dipping and rising as they go away from the body and rising and dipping as they return.

The trigram for An is one yang line on top, a yin line in the middle and a yang line at the bottom. This can imply hardness surrounding softness. For example, in making a push one might find that one is met by strong resistance, yang meets yang. Instead of increasing the power of one's own push, like two stags butting their heads together, one yields, introducing the yin, as it were, from the inside of the trigram. This may cause the aggressive partner to lose balance for a moment, and then, with the yang from the bottom of the trigram, he is made to topple over.

When Push is done, the body moves as a whole, as it does in all Tai Chi movements. The arms do not extend from the action of the triceps muscles alone but are powered from the legs, up the back and into the palms. The arms are simply transmitters. Push is such a committed type of movement that there is danger of losing one's balance forwards and falling through the exuberance of one's own impetuosity! Therefore, care should be exercised in not letting the knee of the leading leg extend beyond the toes. A similar caution can be observed in all movements that go forward.

5. PULL (TSAI)

There are once again several variations in the performance of this action. The trigram for it is a yin line at the base with two yang lines on top. Whatever the style, the movement of Tsai is a pulling one. It has been compared with the posture Needle at Sea Bottom in which the body inclines deeply forward, a rare event in Yang style, and the hands thrust down, but the posture of Lifting Hands or T'i Shou can equally be seen as a prelude to Pull. One can interpret the trigram as beginning at the base with a yin action, when the first grip is taken on the partner's arm, and there is an immediate attempt to detect his or her state of balance and a readiness to yield. At this yin stage, one is ready to release, give way or change direction, should the opportunity for yang not exist. If the conditions are right, then the powerful pull, with yang force incorporating the full weight of the descending body, can be applied.

In the Yang Long Form, Cheng's Short Form and the Long Wu Style Form, the action of Pull can be followed by Shoulder or Elbow strokes, Kao or Chou. This means that should an initial Pull be unsuccessful and the partner draws back, one can follow up with the Elbow or Shoulder strokes to send him on his way. In the Yang and Wu forms, the Needle at Sea Bottom is followed by the posture Fan Penetrates Back, which is a diverting and pushing action, also implying that an initial pull action can be followed by a combined yielding and pushing one. In the pre-arranged Push Hands form of Ta-Lu, the Dance, the posture Tsai plays an important part, and it indicates its importance as a 'fighting' movement.

Pulling may take place downwards or to the side. Whenever and however Pull is used, the whole body weight should be transmitted through the arms. This is one of the hardest lessons for beginners, who almost invariably use arm and shoulder muscle strength. One ought to remember that a body, one's own body, weighs from say 50–100kg. This weight, when applied correctly, uses far less energy to produce a result than an equal weight of effort produced mainly by muscle contraction of the arms. Just imagine a huge pair of scales and in one of the pans a weight of say 55kg. If you weigh 60kg the only thing you have to do to lift that weight is sit in the other pan! If you tried to lift it with your arms and back it would be a completely different experience I imagine – so it is with Pull. Hold the arm and, so to speak, sit down. It is 60kg pulling down one arm.

6. SPLIT (LIEH)

Split is an action like chopping wood and it occurs many times in all forms of Tai Chi. In the form, as distinct from application to combat, There is an opportunity for Split whenever hands and arms descend.

In Push Hands training, it can be used to depress a partner's arm(s) and can be followed by Press, Ward Off or Push. If, for example, in Push Hands, your partner seizes both your upper arms in an attempt to imbalance you forwards or even throw you off balance to his left, you can step out to your right, bring both arms up inside his in a curve and Split his left arm, stepping in between his legs with your left foot and Ward Off to your left. He will fly away! Split, if timed correctly, produces an upward reaction in your partner because he will believe he is being taken down and will resist this, preparing his body for Push or Ward Off from you. Good timing is probably the most important part of this action.

ABOVE SPLIT, WHICH IS USED TO DEPRESS AN OPPONENT'S ARMS, IS A COMMON MOVEMENT IN TAI CHI.

27

The trigram for Split shows a strong yang line at the base and two yin lines on top. This can mean a strong, powerful beginning that upsets the partner, Split downwards, to be followed by a yielding to his reaction upwards leading to another yang action, that of Ward Off, for instance. In trigram interpretation, a strong yang always leads to yin, just as the height of summer leads to a decline to autumn. The movement of the waist, the turning of the waist and pelvis, right or left, is important in Tai Chi and in Split followed by Ward Off, we have a decisive turn right and then left in the example given above. The two steps with the legs, right and left, make this an excellent exercise in combining two of the Eight Gates.

7. ELBOW (CHOU)

Even more yang in the trigram associated with Chou once more leads to yin. Two yang lines at the bottom and one yin line on top indicate a powerful beginning concealed from view. Elbow or elbow stroke is a strong action using all the body weight, with the point of the elbow naturally in line with the solar plexus. In Cheng's form, the elbow is

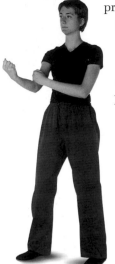

presented to the front with the left hand 'slotted' into the crease of the right arm. In the Chen movement of Elbow Hitting the Heart, the arm is bent or folded horizontally and strikes under the partner's right arm. Yang Cheng-fu's students show Elbow with the left hand held palm out alongside the striking elbow, to protect or deflect. Wu style application of the movement is similar to that of the Chen. This is not an action that lends itself to friendly Push Hands training, unless it is pulled before reaching the target or unless the partner under attack is allowed always to deflect it with his hand. It is too dangerous.

The concealment suggested by the trigram is found in the fact that Elbow is a surprise, close in attack. If your arms are being pushed, it is a simple matter to let the elbow bend and move in towards the partner as he or she comes forward so that the partner 'impales' himself on the elbow point. Elbow turning can also be used to free oneself from an arm or wrist grip. If your partner grips your right wrist with his left hand, you turn your elbow outwards and forwards towards his body, breaking through the 'tiger's mouth' – the space between finger and thumb, the weakest point.

ABOVE THE ELBOW MOVEMENT HAS A POWERFUL BEGINNING, AS IS INDICATED BY THE TWO YANG LINES AT THE BOTTOM OF ITS TRIGRAM.

8. SHOULDER (KAO)

When the hands cannot be used, use the elbow, and when the elbow cannot be used, use the shoulder and when the shoulder cannot be used, use the torso. When the torso cannot be used, think again! Kao or Shoulder is an even closer movement than Elbow and in a sense follows naturally from it. If you attack with Elbow and your partner depresses or turns aside the attack, you simply let your body move in with Shoulder.

In Chen style, this action is done in a very low horse-riding stance. In Yang style, it can be done in a bow stance. In the Wu style, the action begins with an almost bending-double position, ducking under the partner and rising with considerable force to send him off balance. In the Yang version, the Shoulder attack is a direct blow to the front of the body, using legs, waist and back to produce a devastating shock. In Push Hands training, it should be used with caution and placed on the partner's chest to give a pushing action rather than an actual blow.

Its trigram is one yang line on top of two yin lines. This arrangement can suggest the essentially hidden nature of Shoulder. When this technique is used there is no warning as there is in other movements. There is no raising of the hands, only the launching of the body by the legs. Out of this hidden initial action the powerful surprise of the shoulder hit, yang, emerges. However, it is easy to lose balance when performing Shoulder, so the

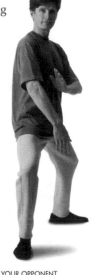

ABOVE YOUR OPPONENT WILL HAVE NO WARNING THAT YOU ARE ABOUT TO USE THE SHOULDER.

29

yin lines can suggest an element of readiness to yield, to take care, to avoid loss of balance and to give up the attack should it seem that the partner is prepared for it. There is a temptation to lean forward too far when doing Shoulder and this invites loss of balance, so that the dictum to keep the spine erect and the centre of gravity low applies here. Obviously exceptions to this posture can occur.

THE FIVE STEPS OF TAI CHI

The Five Steps are so named because of the correspondence that Tai Chi theorists made between the Five Element or Activity theory of Chinese philosophy – namely that everything is composed of metal, wood, water, fire and earth in different proportions – and their own art.

THE FIVE STEPS

The Five Steps of Tai Chi are Advance, Retreat, Look Left, Look Right and Equilibrium.

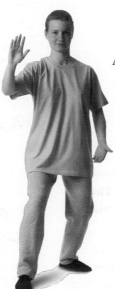

ADVANCE

Associated with Metal. Here Metal 'conquers' or cuts through Wood, or Retreat. When the partner retreats, advance more quickly and send him off balance.

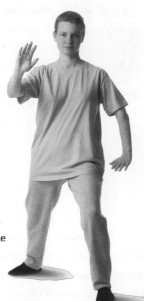

RETREAT

Associated with Wood. Here Wood 'conquers' or upsets Earth, Equilibrium, by pulling and bringing the partner off balance.

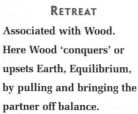

LOOK LEFT

Associated with Water. Here Water 'extinguishes' Fire, Look Right, when for instance a right handed Roll-Back can be upset by a left handed Push leading to a counter move.

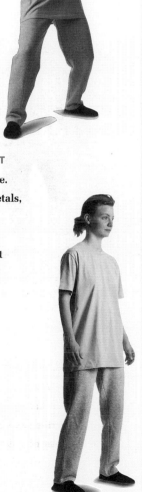

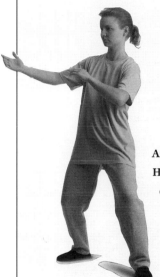

LOOK RIGHT

Associated with Fire. Here fire 'melts' Metals, or Advance, by leading a frontal attack to the right and sending the partner off balance.

EQUILIBRIUM

Associated with Earth. Here Earth 'soaks up' Water, or Look Left, which can mean that sound balance or equilibrium can absorb an attack from the left.

A little reflection, however, shows that Retreat can just as well defeat Advance in actual training, and that any of the other four steps can defeat Earth, Equilibrium if used at the right moment. That is, any step can be defeated by or can defeat any other step depending on circumstances. In the natural world, fire is sometimes extinguished by water, but at other times it boils water out of existence! At other times, a kind of balance between fire and water is maintained by equal proportions of condensation and evaporation. To meet such edifying exceptions, the Five Activities supporters have produced varying cycles of the Activities and cross connections that shore up their ideas. The point is that to try to force one's Tai Chi into conformity with a theory is a mistake. The Five Activities can sometimes be seen as a useful tool, and at other times a disastrous one.

ADDITIONAL POSTURES

As the Yang style of Tai Chi is by far the best known and the most widely performed, and since even the modern Chinese developments in the art are largely based on Yang movements, we shall make it the subject of our discussion. Although there are other postures and movements besides the basic eight and the five steps or directions, all the additional postures contain something of the original 13.

SINGLE WHIP

This is the most distinctive posture of Tai Chi and is traditionally done with the left hand pushing out to the front. The right hand brings the fingers and thumb tips together ,with the wrist bent like the beak of a Crane. Some Tai Chi teachers hold the left hand so that the thumb is bent in, giving the 'tiger's mouth' the appearance of a cobra's open jaws. It is said that Tai Chi movement comes from the actions of a crane and a snake. In Chen and Wu styles, the Single Whip is performed with the legs in a horse-riding stance, the trunk facing out, away from the line of the hand actions. In Yang style, most of the weight is on the front foot with the rear foot at right angles or turned into 45 degrees. The use of Push and Pull can be seen in its action. The general direction of movement in the Yang style is forward, Advance, Metal. The Crane's beak can be used to hook aside an advancing arm, whilst the other hand pushes the chest. My own first teacher told me that the outstretched right arm exerts beneficial pressure on the liver.

LEFT ENTERING INTO THE SINGLE WHIP. THE SINGLE WHIP OCCURS IN ALL TAI CHI STYLES. IT IS PERHAPS THE BEST KNOWN MOVEMENT IN TAI CHI.

33

LIFT HANDS AND PLAY GUITAR

The same posture, but the first is done with the right hand and leg leading and the second with the left leading. In the Wu and Yang styles, the body is erect, with the heel of the leading leg touching the ground, sole raised. The hands resemble the position one would be in when playing a guitar. It has the action Pull implied in it, having seized the partner's arm, and is a retreating movement, Wood.

WHITE CRANE SPREADS ITS WINGS
(ALSO KNOWN AS STORK COOLS ITS WINGS)

A graceful and evocative posture and name. The right hand is raised high to the right like an ascending wing and the left hand lowered to the thigh like a descending one. As a child, I remember hearing the impressive news that a local man had had his arm broken by the beating of a swan's wing and I stayed clear of them thereafter. White Crane is potentially both soft and hard. When a student has reached a sufficient standard of relaxation, then he or she can move the arms rather like wings and produce a kind of undulating, beating effect. In the Wu style, it is performed with a bend and turn of the waist, and bears little resemblance to the upright, graceful movement of the Yang style. The Chen version is closest to the image of a Crane, the arms spreading out one after the other in a low, compact stance. Though conveying the idea of flying, the posture also manages to give an impression of stability, grandeur even, and so one could put it into the category of Earth, Equilibrium. Yang Cheng-fu's own application of the rising hand was to parry or deflect a blow to the head, while the descending had the possibility of parrying a punch or kick to the groin. In Chinese mythology, the Crane is regarded as a symbol of longevity, though this does not seem to have any connection with the name of the posture. In the Yang form, the posture leads into Brush Knee and Twist Step, which is our next movement.

ABOVE THE RIGHT HAND IS LIFTED UPWARDS IN THE WHITE CRANE SPREADS ITS WINGS.

BRUSH KNEE AND TWIST STEP

This is a very common movement that occurs on the left and right sides. It is done in the Chen style, with a high-raised knee followed by a step, and in the Yang style,

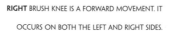

RIGHT BRUSH KNEE IS A FORWARD MOVEMENT. IT OCCURS ON BOTH THE LEFT AND RIGHT SIDES.

with a low, deep step; the Wu version is performed with the characteristic inclination of the trunk forward. Like White Crane, the combined actions of the hands operate at head level and groin or thigh level. Brush Knee contains deflecting but more prominently Push. The direction is forward, Advance, and so it can be equated with Metal.

The modern Combined Tai Chi form has a similar high knee raise like the Chen style demonstrated by Madam Bow-Sim Mark.

STEP FORWARD, DEFLECT DOWNWARD, INTERCEPT AND PUNCH

A long series of connected movements employing several parts of the 13 Postures. In the Wu style, it is done in a small space, with few steps. Chen style uses a similar series of movements done in a very low horse stance pointing to the emphasis in the style on fighting. In the Yang style, which we are using as a reference point here, the student steps forward, as if pursuing a retreating opponent. Since the general direction is forward, we can equate it with Advance, a Metal movement, but it also has actions of Look Left and Look Right. In relation to the Eight Gates, it has the fundamental Split, Ward Off and Push within it in various guises. In spite of this fact, it is a movement that, because of its elongated nature, is less close to the original 13. These all have a compactness, closeness to the body and simplicity that Step Forward lacks. It may be that, in common with the first 13, this series originally consisted of separate movements that were later strung together. Beginners find this movement more difficult than many of the other movements.

AS IF CLOSING A DOOR – CROSS HANDS

In the Yang style, this is a liberating type of movement, opening the chest wide and then pulling in as though closing two sliding doors together. When the closing is completed, the hands cross at the forearms. The movement and the name are very apt. In the Wu style, the action is mainly on pushing rather than pulling together. The

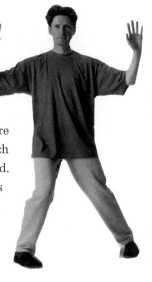

Yang version suggests a position of Equilibrium, Earth, as the arms are brought together, but as the hands reach out to left and right, a Push is indicated. There are several applications of this Door movement, such as pushing aside, scooping up a leg, deflecting an arm and so forth. It is one of the more versatile actions of Tai Chi. When the arms cross, there is a strong impression of balance and solidity.

36

FIST UNDER ELBOW –
PUNCH UNDER ELBOW

In all styles, the basic position of the clenched fist of one hand under the bent elbow of the other is found. The lead in to this movement, in the Yang form, is one of whirling left and right, and this gives a very good example of using the waist to move the arms. This right and left turn hints at both Fire and Water but the movement also shows a type of Roll-Back and Push action, conveying several facets of the original 13. The final recognized posture also has strong equilibrium.

EMBRACE TIGER AND
RETURN TO MOUNTAIN

An evocative name of a Yang style movement that has a strong Push, Look Right and then Retreat; Fire and Wood. The Return includes a kind of Roll-Back or Pull, depending on exactly how it is performed. In all Tai Chi movements, the weight is transferred from one leg to the other in rhythmic sequence and so Equilibrium, Earth, can be said to appear in all as the weight shifts. In some cases, the equilibrium is centrally maintained, but in others it is only passing. In the Five Activities theory, the Earth is placed at the centre through which all directions pass, so one can say that, in this respect, the Five Activities theory is relevant to all the postures.

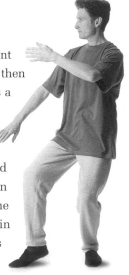

ABOVE THIS IS A DYNAMIC POSTURE, INVOLVING A STRONG FORWARD MOVEMENT.

STEP BACK TO DRIVE MONKEY AWAY

This movement contains a strong, retreating Wood phase or activity. In all styles where it is used, there is a Push with one hand and a Pull with the other combined with a low stance. The rear leg as one steps back takes a lot of the weight, and the thigh muscles are considerably exercised, as beginners frequently testify. Tai Chi teacher Yang Jwing-ming in Boston shows this movement with a strong forward kick with the front leg, a use of the posture that is quite acceptable though not done in the form by most Yang style students.

LEFT THE STEP BACK TO DRIVE MONKEY AWAY POSTURE CAN BE VERY TIRING ON THE THIGH MUSCLES.

DIAGONAL FLYING POSTURE

One of the most pleasing actions of the Yang form, spreading the arms wide, one high, one low and opening the chest wide after holding a ball and sinking the chest prior to performing it. Sometimes one feels with this movement that one really is going to fly. The nearest of the original 13 to this movement would be Ward Off with the leading, rising arm, though the resemblance is not close. One could associate Diagonal Flying with Advance, Look Right or even Equilibrium. I, myself, would choose Advance, Metal. It can be used to strike an opponent with the top edge of the rising forearm and perhaps send him backwards over the leading leg.

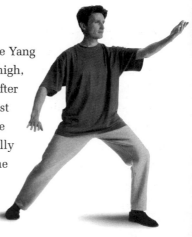

ABOVE DIAGONAL FLYING IS A BOLD, OPEN AND ENERGETIC POSTURE.

FAN PENETRATES BACK

Was this the iron war fan or the poisoned barbed fan? Whatever the origin of this picturesquely named movement, it is very enjoyable to do. The right arm rises to the side of the head and the left pushes up and forwards. One can experience the rib cage expanding and the whole torso opening, as the weight is transferred onto the front leg. Both the Wu and Yang style versions have a certain similarity, with deflecting and

LEFT FAN PENETRATES BACK IS A VERY ENJOYABLE POSTURE, IMPARTING BOTH STRENGTH AND ENERGY.

pushing contained within them. Though the movement has a turn right or left, Fire and Water, the obviously related movement is one of Advance, Metal. Yang Cheng-fu shows the leading hand or palm hitting and the rear rising hand parrying or seizing. He describes the overall positions of the arms as like a bracket, which is a fair comparison. Beginners often place the rear hand too low down and close to the head. This would be useless in parrying a blow to the head so both for exercise and application, it should be well clear of the top of the head and out to the side. If the form is done in this way, then there will be plenty of reserve distance in the action when it comes to defending the head.

WAVE HANDS LIKE (IN) CLOUDS – CLOUD-LIKE HANDS

Long, elongated or circular clouds, depending on teacher and style. If marooned on a desert island and permitted to take only one movement with them, Cloud Hands would be the choice of many Tai Chi students. I think it would be mine. Cloud Hands is a sort of self-contained series of similar movements performed to the left and right sides alternately with small sideways steps. It has Fire, Water and Earth. The arms and hands describe circles across the level of the throat and lower abdomen, which intersect like clouds in the sky. It would be nearer the truth to say that these circles are more like parabolas but sometimes the temptation to make them completely circular is very strong. Wu and Yang styles differ in the way Cloud Hands is performed and the Chen style shows a cross-over step that is very rare in Tai Chi, though often found in other Chinese martial arts; perhaps a pointer to some of the Chen origins. Though the Chen and Wu actions

39

LEFT CLOUD-LIKE HANDS MOVES FROM SIDE

TO SIDE IN A SERIES OF SMALL STEPS.

have their strong points they do not have the same aesthetic satisfaction in them as the Yang action. With a little imagination one can see all of the first six actions of the Eight Gates in Cloud Hands.

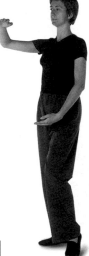

HIGH PAT ON HORSE – STEP UP TO EXAMINE HORSE

Clearly one name was given by an animal lover and the other by a horse doctor! In direction and action, this one is similar to Drive Monkey Away but has a different application. Yang Cheng-fu shows the lower hand depressing a punch and the high hand striking to the face at the same time, and the stance is higher. A retreating, Wood, motion, High Pat is sometimes seen very low in the Yang style.

LEFT HIGH PAT ON HORSE IS A RETREATING POSTURE.

KICKS – SEPARATE RIGHT FOOT, ETC.

Several versions of kicking actions occur in Tai Chi; some of them combined with high leaps, as in Chen style. In general, these are not strongly emphasized in training, especially in Yang style. As a rule one can say that a leg that bears little weight in a posture is potentially a kicking leg, a leg used to block a kick or a leg used to sweep away an opponent's leg. Kicks are usually accompanied by a separation of the arms

RIGHT THE SEPARATE RIGHT FOOT POSTURE

HELPS TO DEVELOP BALANCE.

to the sides or diagonally. The height of kicks is usually limited to the waist in the form training, but obviously a kick can rise if necessary to a higher point. Students need to have a reasonable sense of balance to kick, and in some cases must be able to swivel round on one leg, keep the balance and then kick, all in one unbroken flow. Arguments can be brought to place kicks in any of the Five Activities categories.

STRIKE TIGER - TAME TIGER

Of all the postures of Tai Chi, this one most closely resembles movements akin to those of the Shaolin or hard-style schools. One hand is raised in a fist to protect the face and the other lowered in a fist to protect the abdomen and groin. In the Chen style, it resembles a Karate movement. A similar posture is shown in Chinese and Korean temple guardians, those ancient stone statues or reliefs positioned near the temple entrances, their faces frozen in a ferocious glare to warn off intruders. It is a firm, stable posture reminding one of Equilibrium, Earth. It seems to say that no one will shift me from this position, not

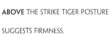

ABOVE THE STRIKE TIGER POSTURE SUGGESTS FIRMNESS.

even a tiger! All Yang Cheng-fu's descendants seem to have used the translation given above as the name of this posture but another has been given and attributed to him – Hiding Tiger Reveals His Face. Perhaps as the hands rise and fall the face of the tiger is seen emerging between them?

STRIKE WITH BOTH FISTS

This is a pleasing movement for the back muscles. I remember learning this movement a long time ago and can still recall the pleasure it gave me to take the arms back and down to the sides,

41

outwards, upwards and forwards. Both arms move together and the thumb edges of both fists strike an opponent on both temples at the same time. It is an Advance, Metal action with no apparent connection with any of the Eight Gates.

PARTING WILD HORSE MANE

This is a free and open movement reminiscent of Diagonal Flying but not quite as open as that. There are several variations within the Yang style but basically one hand rises, palm up, level with the throat and the other hand descends to the thigh. It can be a strike to the neck, a parry, a pull – several things at once. Its overall action is one of Advance and so Metal.

There are many small movements within the Tai Chi – little turns, loops and undulations of the body that cannot properly be described in words. They need a good video or a teacher. Beginners cannot be expected to appreciate them all at once, and this may be why, when the modern 24 Step Peking Form was produced, all the intermediate movements that connect the postures together were taught as if they were postures in themselves. Such an approach leads to a good appreciation of the final position for each posture. For instance, in Part Wild Horse Mane, the intermediate posture shows a 45 degree outward turn to the final direction, then a step forward and then a step into the final direction. This introduces Water, if turning Left, or Fire if turning Right, followed in both cases by Advance, Metal. When we come to look at the tentative table drawn up later in this chapter, we shall find Metal featuring very prominently in it.

FAIR LADY WORKS WITH SHUTTLES –
JADE GIRL WORKS AT SHUTTLES

Both arms are raised above shoulder level in this posture, as in Fan Penetrates Back. It is not common to find the arms raised high in Tai Chi, certainly not in the original 13 Postures. Critics might say that it leaves the body unprotected against kicks, that it lifts the centre of gravity and so on. But on the other hand, if the head is to be protected, the hands must rise and, from an exercise point of view, there are only a small number of ways to exercise the shoulders without doing so.

Fair Lady is an advancing movement, Metal, but may be done to Left or Right, Water or Fire. It is closer to Push and Ward Off than to any of the other Eight Gates. In Yang forms, it is done to the four minor compass directions with a strong turning in of the leading foot to change direction and to shift the weight. Beginners often find this intermediate movement difficult as, at first, they cannot turn in sufficiently. These movements are reminiscent of a movement found in Pa-kua, Eight Trigram Boxing, in which the arms encircle the body, protecting it as a turning movement is made. During this same sequence of intermediate movements, the balance is at greater risk than usual; so when doing them, care should be taken to keep the centre of gravity down to counteract this.

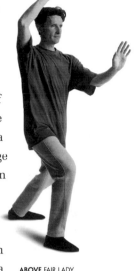

ABOVE FAIR LADY WORKS WITH SHUTTLE REQUIRES FLEXIBILITY AND GOOD BALANCE.

43

GOLDEN ROOSTER STANDS ON ONE LEG

A radical departure from all that has gone before, with a high posture using one leg for support and the other thigh raised to a horizontal position. The action can be used for striking an opponent in the groin with the raised knee, and hitting him under the chin with the open raised palm. One can read this posture as Equilibrium, Earth, since balance is an essential part of it.

LEFT THE GOLDEN ROOSTER STANDS ON ONE LEG POSTURE DEVELOPS BALANCE AND POISE.

SINGLE WHIP SQUATTING DOWN – SNAKE CREEPS DOWN

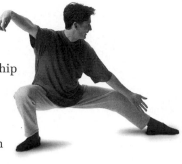

This posture is like the Single Whip posture except that in doing it one squats down on the rear leg and shifts weight back on to the front leg. The front hand protects the groin and then moves out to attack the opponent in the groin. This is a difficult posture to do; flexibility is the order of the day, and strong legs. Approach it with caution.

ABOVE SINGLE WHIP SQUATTING STRENGTHENS THE LEGS AND OPENS THE PELVIC AND HIP REGIONS.

WHITE SNAKE PUTS OUT TONGUE

A posture using one hand snaking out over the other, and with the pointed fingers hitting a soft or vulnerable part of the body such as throat or eyes. It is an Advance, and so a Metal movement.

STEP UP TO THE SEVEN STARS

In the Yang forms, this is a movement that usually follows Snake Creeps Down, using both fists crossed at the wrists. It can be seen as two successive punches or a blocking action using the crossed wrists. This too is an Advance or Metal action.

STEP BACK (RETREAT) TO RIDE THE TIGER

This is a Retreat, Wood, movement that in some ways resembles White Crane.

LEFT AS ITS NAME SUGGESTS, STEP BACK TO RIDE THE TIGER, IS A RETREAT MOVEMENT

TURN BODY AND SWEEP LOTUS LEG

The only spinning action of Yang style. The weight is taken on the right foot and one spins to the right through 360 degrees. To put the left foot down, swing the right foot out and up to the left and then across the body to the right, brushing the outstretched hands with the foot. A posture not really related to any of the 13, and so hard to place. The right leg is usually shown as a sweeping kick to the body of the opponent.

In Chen style, leaping and kicking in the air is not uncommon, and it may be that Sweep Lotus is one of the vestiges of this type of action remaining in the Yang style. From a physical point of view it is hard to generate power in a kick that travels in this particular direction.

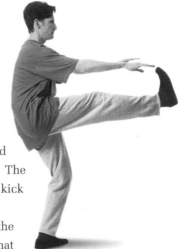

ABOVE THE LEG IS EXTENDED AND SWEPT ACROSS THE FRONT OF THE BODY IN A FAST KICK.

BEND THE BOW AND SHOOT THE TIGER

A posture with several variations in the Yang style alone and one that I have learned and learned again to perform in different ways. The posture looks as though you are making two punching actions, one of which is head height and the other chest height. The relationship of the hands is such that you might be holding and bending a bow with them. Yang Cheng-fu says that

RIGHT IN BEND THE BOW AND SHOOT THE TIGER, ONE HAND IS HELD AT HEAD HEIGHT, WHILE THE OTHER IS AT CHEST HEIGHT.

this action is meant to strike the opponent in the chest.

NEEDLE AT SEA BOTTOM

A unique movement in Tai Chi in which the body bends low to the front, sometimes with the left palm and fingers touching the pulse of the right hand as in Press. It can be interpreted as a strong, pulling down action, and, as it is followed in the Yang forms with the action of Fan Penetrates Back, it can also be an initial upsetting movement to bring a partner off balance forward, producing a backward reaction that Fan can turn into a backward fall.

ANALYZING THE MOVEMENTS

It is interesting to analyse the movements of the Yang style Long Form in terms of the frequency of the Eight Gates or Postures and the Five Activities combined with other aspects of life such as the organs of the body as found in Chinese traditional medicine (*see* pp.48–49). Such an analysis should be seen merely as an example of a Chinese way of looking at different phenomena and relating them, and not as a definitive version. Of the Five activities we have in the table:

81 postures correspond to Metal – West – Lungs – Large Intestine
25 postures correspond to Wood – East – Liver – Gall Bladder
24 postures correspond to Earth – Centre – Spleen – Stomach

Then merely a sprinkling of seven mingled directions, activities and body organs from the two areas of Fire and Water. Remember that the directions in this case have nothing to do with the directions taken in the form, but with the correspondences made in Tai Chi and medical theory. On the face of it, then, there are approximately three times the number of Metal associated postures as there are of Wood or Earth postures taken on their own; and a ratio of three to two if taken in combination with one another. Here we must look at the intermediate movements and the smaller movements, which are not apparent until you do the forms for yourself.

It was pointed out earlier that the Centre, Equilibrium, Earth activity is constantly being passed through, and that throughout the form, the activity of Look Left and Right appears in the form repeatedly, in intermediate movements. If we count these lesser movements then the balance of activities changes. But taking the table as it stands, we find a largely yang sequence of movements, partly balanced by yin movements. This seems to upset the idea of Tai Chi as a yin type of exercise.

This calls into question for Western Tai Chi students the widely held Western view of Tai Chi as a yin form of exercise (remember that the Chen style, with its emphasis on fighting, agility and power was the father of the modern art of Yang style). One of my own theories, is that during the 1960s and 1970s when the Hippie movement was in full swing, many Western young people were looking for an experience that was gentle and non-aggressive. An intellectually weak grasp of Taoist philosophy and Tai Chi seems to indicate that these two aspects of Chinese culture fit that kind of bill. My own opinion is that they do not.

47

A further reason for the popularity of the mainly yin view of Tai Chi is the beneficial effect it can have on stress. Many people associated yin with relaxation and yang with tension. This too is a mistake. Yin can be tense and yang relaxed. We shall see later that the yin-yang theory proposes that when any condition reaches an extreme it has to change and extreme yin or yang in the human body falls into that category. A third reason for the yin view is the very great difficulty there is in combining yin and yang equally in Tai Chi performance, especially in

LEFT YIN YANG SYMBOL. THE ART OF TAI CHI CONTAINS BOTH YIN AND YANG, FOR THERE CANNOT BE ONE WITHOUT THE OTHER.

YANG STYLE LONG FORM – ANALYSIS

	Times Used	Dominant Phrase	Direction	Yin Organ	Yang Organ
Beginning	1	Earth	Centre	spleen	stomach
Ward Off	11	Metal	West	lungs	large intestine
Roll-Back	8	Wood	East	liver	gall bladder
Press	8	Metal	West	lungs	large intestine
Push	8	Metal	West	lungs	large intestine
Single Whip	11	Metal	West	lungs	large intestine
Lift Hands	5	Wood	East	liver	gall bladder
White Crane	3	Earth	Centre	spleen	stomach
Brush Knee	10	Metal	West	lungs	large intestine
Step, Deflect	5	Metal	West	lungs	large intestine
Close Door	3	Earth	Centre	kidneys/spleen/heart	bladder/stomach/small intestine
Cross Hands	1	Earth	Centre	kidneys/spleen/heart	bladder/stomach/small intestine
Embrace Tiger	2	Fire/Water	North/South	kidneys/heart	bladder/small intestine
Punch Elbow	1	Earth	Centre	spleen	stomach
Chop	4	Metal	West	lungs	large intestine

Posture	No.	Element	Direction	Organ	Organ
Monkey	7	Wood	East	liver	gall bladder
Diagonal	2	Metal	West	lungs	large intestine
Needle	2	Wood	East	liver	gall bladder
Fan Back	2	Metal	West	lungs	large intestine
Wave Hands	14	Earth	Centre	spleen	stomach
Pat Horse	2	Wood	East	liver	gall bladder
Kicks	10	Metal	West	lungs	large intestine
Punch Down	2	Metal	West	lungs	large intestine
Tame Tiger	2	Earth	Centre	spleen	stomach
Both Fists	1	Metal	West	lungs	large intestine
Horse Mane	3	Metal	West	lungs	large intestine
Fair Lady	4	Metal/Water/Fire	West/North/South	lungs/kidneys/heart	large intestine/bladder/small intestine
Snake Creeps	2	Metal	West	lungs	large intestine
Golden Rooster	2	Earth	Centre	spleen	stomach
White Snake	1	Metal	West	lungs	large intestine
Seven Stars	1	Metal	West	lungs	large intestine
Ride Tiger	1	Wood	East	liver	gall bladder
Bend Bow	1	Fire/Metal	South/West	heart/lungs	small intestine/large intestine

THIS TABLE SHOULD BE READ BEARING IN MIND TEXTUAL REFERENCES TO INTERMEDIATE MOVEMENTS.

Yang Style Long Form Postures

The following is a list of the postures in the Yang style Long Form with some abbreviated names. If a posture is done more than once in a sequence, this is shown by a multiplication sign and the number of times it occurs, for example, Monkey x 5. Read down each column beginning at the left hand side of the page.

Beginning	White Crane
Ward Off Left	Brush Knee
Ward Off Right	Needle Sea Bottom
Roll-Back	Fan Penetrates Back
Press	Turn and Chop
Push	Step Forward
Single Whip	Ward Off
Lift Hands	Roll-Back
White Crane	Press
Brush Knee x 5	Push
Play Guitar x 2	Single Whip
Step Forward	Wave Hands Clouds x 5
Closing Door	Single Whip
Embrace Tiger	High Pat Horse
Ward Off	Kicks x 3
Roll-Back	Brush Knee x 2
Press	Punch
Push	Turn and Chop
Single Whip	Step Forward
Punch Elbow	Kick
Monkey x 5	Tame Tiger x 2
Diagonal Flying	Kick
Lift Hands	Strike Both Fists

Kicks x 3

Chop

Step Forward

Closing Door

Embrace Tiger

Ward Off

Roll-Back

Press

Push

Single Whip

Part Horse Mane x 3

Ward Off Left

Ward Off Right

Roll-Back

Press

Push

Single Whip

Fair Lady x 4

Ward Off Left

Ward Off Right

Roll-Back

Press

Push

Single Whip

Wave Hands Clouds x 5

Single Whip

Snake Creeps

Golden Rooster x 2

Monkey x 2

Diagonal Flying

Lift Hands

White Crane

Brush Knee

Needle Sea Bottom

Fan Penetrates Back

White Snake Tongue

Step Forward

Ward Off

Roll-Back

Press

Push

Single Whip

Wave Hands Clouds x 5

Single Whip

High Pat Horse

Cross Hands

Kick

Brush Knee

Punch

Ward Off

Roll-Back

Press

Push

Single Whip

Seven Stars

Ride Tiger

Kick

Bend Bow

Chop

Step Forward

Closing Door

Conclusion

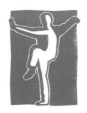

PUSH HANDS AND COMBAT

CHAPTER THREE

When a Tai Chi student has been learning the form for some time, the teacher will introduce training in Push Hands (Tui Shou) and later on training in the combat use of the movements (San Shou). Push Hands is a very formal method of training, in which two students stand facing one another and rest their hands on one another's arms. They then push and yield alternately using a variety of methods found in the form, such as Push, Roll-Back, Press, Ward Off and so on.

At first this is done without moving the feet. The aim here is to accustom them to apply force and yield to force using only the arms, torso and fixed legs. Later, Push Hands with steps is introduced, and there are also formal or pre-arranged

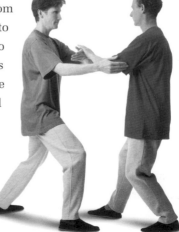

RIGHT IN PUSH HANDS, STUDENTS TAKE IT IN TURNS TO PUSH AND TO YIELD.

movements in this phase. One of the more elaborate training methods is called the Dance, Ta-Lu. It is a 'dance' in the sense that students move together in certain directions, their hands always in contact in a variety of ways.

The degree of force, speed and movement used in any class will depend on the attitude of the teacher and proficiency of the students. Whatever variations in action may be permitted in the class, the aim is the same. This is to relax the body, be sensitive to the incoming force such as a push, not to give way to aggressive emotions, and learn to make maximum use of one's own and one's partner's bodyweight.

Inevitably, a competitive element appears in Push Hands, but overall the student tries to dissipate this by concentrating on the other factors mentioned above. One student tries to keep his balance as the other tries to make him lose it, and then the roles are reversed.

Some Tai Chi classes do not do Push Hands at all. But, in my opinion, without it Tai Chi development is arrested. When a student does only the solo forms, it is possible to dream that balance is good, relaxation is sound and posture is correct; in short that everything is fine. However, when another student lays his or her hands on you and gives you a push, all these assumptions are tested.

53

An Internal Martial Art

This struggle for inner calm and non-attachment is one of the reasons why Tai Chi is called an internal martial art. If the inside and the outside do not correspond, then the Tai Chi will not be good. The external martial arts harness aggression, fearsome expressions, muscle power and hardness. The internal need some strength too, but they also look for a calm interior, a willingness to be sensitive to the other and a desire to explore and learn. Without this the balance is lost.

Internal martial arts are also sometimes called soft. This has led some students to interpret soft to mean floppy or weak; but this is a mistake. Soft means something that results from having the right internal/external balance. It is a kind of resilience, like the softness of rubber, yielding yet springing back into shape. Since it is contrary to our usual behaviour to be like this, training in Push Hands is a much greater test of one's Tai Chi than solo form training. It is a lifelong study, extending outside the Tai Chi class itself.

This turning of the attention inside oneself is found in Taoist, Ch'an Buddhist and Zen Buddhist teachings, among others. An excellent illustration comes from a letter written in the 17th century by Takuan, the famous abbot of a Zen monastery, Daitokuji, in Kyoto, Japan, to a swordsman, Yagyu Tajima No Kami Munenori:

> '*Have no intention to counterattack him in response to his threatening move, cherish no calculating thoughts whatever. You simply perceive the opponent's move, you do not allow your mind to 'stop' with it, you move on just as you are toward the opponent and make use of his attack to turn it on to himself... Kwannon Bosatsu (Avaloketisvara) is sometimes represented with one thousand arms, each holding a different instrument. If his mind 'stops' with the use, for instance, of a bow, all the other arms, nine hundred and ninety-nine in number, will be of no use whatever. It is only because of his mind not 'stopping' with the use of one arm but moving from one instrument to another that all his arms prove useful with the utmost degree of efficiency.'*
> (D T Suzuki, Zen and Japanese Culture.)

The above illustrates clearly the principle of not fixing, 'freezing' or tensing as a result of the desire to win at all costs. Constant and fluid motion is needed so that the partner in Push Hands has no solid point on which to rest his or her arms to give a strong push.

TAI CHI COMBAT

Like everything else, Push Hands can turn into a habit, in the sense that a given routine with a regular partner can lull both into a happy, sleeping state in which nothing ever changes. This is why Push Hands should be varied and why it should be extended into combat-type training sessions.

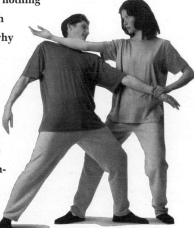

In this type of session there is not only pushing but gripping and pulling, which brings Tai Chi nearer to the Chinese martial art of Chin-na or the art of seizing. This is not outside the traditions of Tai Chi. Yang Cheng-fu, Cheng Man-ch'ing and many other Tai Chi masters made routine use of techniques outside the purely pushing

ABOVE TAI CHI COMBAT IS A REAL TEST OF ONE'S SKILL, SENSITIVITY AND ATTITUDE.

field. In theory, one should be able to elude a grip or pull without losing one's balance. Few people can, but the aim is still there, drawing one on to greater efforts. There is always at least one unguarded moment when the grip of a partner is weaker, and this is the moment to escape from it.

The weight of the body itself is a factor that many students overlook. We are so accustomed to using only our muscles to accomplish something that our weight is forgotten. Even a person weighing only 50 kilograms is able to move that weight against or away from a partner. If he or she finds the right way to do this, then the power of a movement can be greatly increased.

55

FIXED STEP PUSH HANDS

Push Hands without moving the feet is generally translated as Fixed Step Push Hands. If we look at the performance of Push Hands with the steps excluded, we find that most of the movements are carried out in the Bow Stance – right or left foot forward carrying most of the weight, knee bent and the rear leg almost straight. When the weight is shifted on to the back leg, a kind of reverse of the Bow Stance, sometimes called Empty Stance, that leg carries most of the weight and the front leg is slightly bent. Bow Stance is used for the Push, Ward Off and Press advancing movements and the Empty Step for Roll-Back and retreating movements. Pushing and yielding, advancing and retreating, trace a pattern of curves, although pushing tends at the beginning to be straight. A good rule of thumb is to say that to reduce the force of a push in a straight line, you lead it into a curve, and to counteract the effect of a yielding curve, you reintroduce a straight line. To do this you can have no preconceived ideas since you never know in advance what will happen. Pushing in the early stages is done by resting one hand on the wrist of a partner and the other on the elbow, thus preventing a possible punch or elbow blow. Furthermore, by controlling the elbow you have a certain amount of leverage directly on the trunk of your partner through his upper arm, rather like the manoeuvrable handle on a heavy trolley. Later this hand position can be changed to pushing on the shoulder, the chest, the hips and even the knees. In general, Push Hands does not

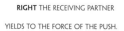

RIGHT THE RECEIVING PARTNER
YIELDS TO THE FORCE OF THE PUSH.

include the head since it could cause injury to the cervical vertebrae in the neck. Other parts of the body are also used to push with; the elbow, the shoulder, the side of the body, even the buttocks! The last three are for very close-in work.

The artificial restriction on leg movement in the Fixed Step Push Hands makes it imperative that students find a way to let the body give way on its own. The bending of the knees can help. but also the turning of the hips and the sinking of the chest are needed. Also, the free movement of the shoulder blade, the scapula, can greatly assist the free movement of the arm. The next stage is to allow one or two

THE TA-LU

The Ta-lu varies from club to club but it is always a series of pre-arranged steps and movements involving gripping, pulling and pushing, and escaping from gripping, yielding to pulling and pushing. For example, student A will push towards the South. Student B will yield to the push and step back, maybe gripping A by one arm and pull him, at the same time stepping back at right angles, to East or West. Student A yields to the pull, steps after student B and maybe attacks with Shoulder. Student B diverts the Shoulder attack and pushes and so on.

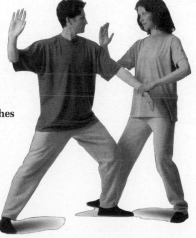

RIGHT TA-LU SHOWS STUDENTS HOW TO KEEP THEIR BALANCE IN MOVEMENT.

steps backwards and forwards so that students get used to the idea of moving the feet and at the same time keeping their arms in contact with the partner's arms. Once a student is used to moving one or two steps, the next stage, the Ta-lu, or Dance, can be introduced (*see* p.57). The next stages will depend very much on the teacher. He may teach a range of other applications of Tai Chi movements or he may gradually escalate the tempo and strength of the training until the level of Tai Chi Combat is reached.

Not everyone who comes to Tai Chi likes Push Hands. Some people want only the calming and relaxing effects of doing the forms. If a person's resistance to being taught Push Hands is strong, then the teacher should respect it, because a student will not make much progress if he or she harbours feelings of resentment as a result of being compelled to do something that is disliked. My own contact with Push Hands was at first sporadic. It seemed to me to be at odds with the fundamentals of Tai Chi, which I saw as primarily yin, yielding. Over the years my attitude changed. I began to see it as a discipline of non-aggression and a means of using strong action without the emotional intent to injure. When I began to teach, it brought me a great deal of satisfaction to see men and women, some of them big and strong, learn to check the desire to win in favour of learning something about the interplay of yin and yang.

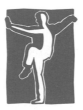

TAI CHI WEAPONS

CHAPTER FOUR

In the Chinese martial arts tradition, skill with a weapon has always been placed on a higher level than skill with the empty hand. This is partly because more skill is required to wield a weapon, and partly because in the past a nobleman or gentleman would not as a rule 'stoop' to bare first fighting. Bodyguards were employed to deal with such distasteful things.

Today this attitude has changed in the sense that there is no longer a class distinction concerning weapons. In the mainland Chinese Wushu (martial arts) training syllabus, the students are introduced to empty hand forms first and to weapons later; purely on a basis of the degree of difficulty. Many of the hand positions, stances and body movements of unarmed forms are used in the weapons forms and a beginner is better served by being taught the former first. Once the body is trained then, when the weapons arc taken up, a student can concentrate his attention on the intricacies of the sword, spear or pole techniques without having to think about the basic factors.

Not all teachers teach the same weapons in Tai Chi. However, a common selection from the vast array of Wushu arms include the Jen, a classical double-edged straight sword; the Dao (Big Knife), a single-edged curved sword resembling what we in the West would call a scimitar; the Ch'iang, spear; and sometimes a long type of halberd.

THE SWORD

The Tai Chi sword varies in length and ideally should suit the height and weight of the user. The swords available today include antique swords, modern swords of spring steel, alloy swords, swords composed of two laminated metal strips and wooden swords.

A right-handed student holds the sword mainly in that hand, but at the beginning of most sword forms it is held by the left hand using a reverse grip. This means that the flat of the blade runs up along the left arm pointing towards and beyond the armpit and shoulder. After a few movements of the form, the left hand places the handle in the open right palm. Then the left hand takes on a particular shape. This consists of the index finger and middle finger held straight in line with the palm and the remaining two fingers being folded across the palm with the thumb pressed down on top of them. This hand formation is known as the sword charm, the sword amulet or the helper of the secret sword. In sword form theory, this sword charm is supposed to conduct vital energy, Chi, into the right sword arm at the point of the pulse, the wrist, during many of the movements of the form. Chi is said to flow from the two pointing fingers and into the acupuncture channels. The pressure of the sword charm can also help in the technique in which the sword tip is moved in a circle. The tips of the pointing fingers press down on the end of the sword handle to assist this

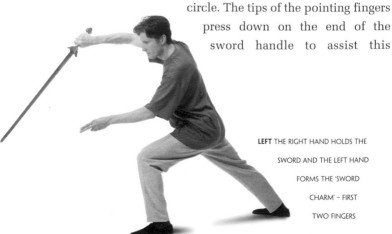

LEFT THE RIGHT HAND HOLDS THE SWORD AND THE LEFT HAND FORMS THE 'SWORD CHARM' – FIRST TWO FINGERS

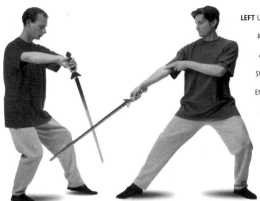

LEFT USING A TAI CHI SWORD REQUIRES CONSIDERABLE SKILL AND DEFT FOOTWORK. THE SWORD FORM WILL ALSO ENHANCE MENTAL ALERTNESS AND AGILITY.

action. Furthermore, since the Tai Chi sword is wielded mainly by one arm and therefore puts more of a demand on the muscles of the right side of the trunk, the sword charm position and its movement in harmony with the sword arm helps to activate and use the left side of the body, giving a certain degree of energy balance.

The movement of the body during a sword form should be lithe, fluid and lively. This applies when the form in question is quick. When the form is slow, calm and measured, as in some versions of the Yang style sword form that follow the same pace as the Long Form, students are taught to make their movements correspond as much as possible to the feeling of that empty hand form.

A key point in sword use is a strong and flexible wrist and elbow. The sense of balance needs to be more highly developed than in the empty hand form since the momentum of the blade as it sweeps and cuts tends to pull the body out of alignment.

STANCES AND ACTIONS

The Yang family sword form requires the expenditure of much more energy than the empty hand form. This is not just because a student is holding a weapon but because there is much more activity in it. This may be because the sword form is closer to the original Chen style with its greater emphasis on varied movement

61

and changes in tempo. Video tapes of Chen style from Taiwan and mainland China confirm this theory.

The chief stance of the form is the Bow Stance, sometimes called the archery stance, taken rather wide and deep, weight on the front leg as in the empty hand form. Some instructors, mainly from the Shaolin or hard-style schools of Kung Fu, say that in this stance the weight is evenly distributed on both legs. The only way to manage this is for the bent front leg to push back as it were against the pelvis and transfer force back on to the rear leg. This is not the way it is done in Tai Chi.

Another stance that is used in the sword form is the tip stance or T-stance with the weight on the rear leg and the front leg resting on the ball of the foot or toes, heel slightly raised. The stance, which can be seen in a sense as the reverse of the Bow Stance, is the Waist Drawn Back stance or Empty Stance, again with weight on the rear leg but with the whole of the sole of the front foot touching the ground. The Horse Riding Stance, like a person sitting on a large horse, has the feet spread wide apart, more or less parallel, and this stance occurs a few times in the sword form. The stance with one leg raised, thigh more or less parallel with the floor, does not seem to have been given a name but it could safely be called a Crane Stance; it also appears several times in the sword form.

The remaining noteworthy stance is assumed by bending the rear leg deeply, almost a squat, and the front leg sliding forward. It is similar to the stance for Snake Creeps Down or Single Whip Squatting Down in the empty hand form. The stance is sometimes called the Sliding Stance.

THE DAO

The Dao or scimitar, or Big Knife as it is sometimes called, is about one metre long; curved, sharp along one edge and the blunt edge or back some 12mm thick. Dr Tseng Ju-pai records that blades should not be swung so that the cutting edge cross the fontanel, the place on the top of the skull where the bones meet. This point, approximately in the middle of the head, is traditionally thought of as the point through which a person's spiritual energy connects with heaven. However, if the blunt edge of the Dao is swung back over this point, this is acceptable since it does not have the power to cut through spiritual energy.

It is believed that the Dao originated in the Bronze Age. Stories are told of how the Dao was used during the Chinese war with the Japanese in hand-to-hand combat.

Many of the techniques of the Dao involve a slashing movement. The nature of the Dao's use is very fierce, like a tiger, and the use of the weapon in the Yang family form does not show the weapon off to its best advantage. However, Madam Bow-Sim Mark's demonstration of the Dao, as found in the modern Wushu training syllabus, shows its great dynamic potential. Speaking in general, it is true to say that greater physical fitness and agility is needed to use the Dao well than to wield the Jen well.

63

THE SPEAR

The spear, Ch'iang, varies in length from about two to three metres. The haft, whatever wood is used, should be pliable and resilient for Tai Chi. A rigid type of wood is not suitable. The head of the spear is roughly diamond shape with a taper to a point. Almost invariably, a bundle of tassels is tied around the place where the head is fixed to the shaft. Frequently, horse mane or tail hair is used and dyed red. When a student shakes the spear during training, the vibration of the hair indicates something about the quality of his Chi and his muscular strength. It is also said that the hair absorbs blood, and this may explain the use of red dye to signify the colour that it would become in battle.

If the use of the Dao is comparatively rare, then use of the spear is rarer still. Dr Tseng Ju-pai was taught two uses of the spear by Yang Cheng-fu. The first he called unilateral drill and the second bilateral drill. The unilateral drill consisted mainly of shaking the spear. This action of shaking is connected with the pliability of the wood used for the haft of the spear. When the weapon is shaken by an expert, you can see the energy travelling down the vibrating wood to the point. If the wood were dense and rigid and, so to speak, insensitive to the movement, it would not convey this vibration, and the user would not be able to transmit his energy to the point in quite the same way. Tai Chi shaking of the spear would be impossible.

In the bilateral drill there are 13 actions of attack and defence grouped in four categories. These are: tenacity, rebound, tenacity and rebound combined and entanglement. Tenacity echoes the idea of Push Hands training where one tries to remain in contact with one's partner. Rebound contains the notion of using the opponent's energy to move one's own weapon. Tenacity and rebound studies the combination of the first two. Entanglement involves wrapping one's own spear around the spear of the partner, although this notion cannot be carried too far and usually means advancing with a circling action with the two spears in contact. The spear point in this action of Entanglement moves in a spiral or series of circles, reminiscent of the basic techniques of the Western fencing foil. Sometimes the spear, held in the right hand, is thrust through the lightly clenched palm of the left hand between the first finger and the thumb. The movement is comparable with sliding a snooker cue over the hand.

A final word about weapons training – they need a lot of space. For empty hand forms a relatively small area can be used for training but when wielding a sword or scimitar, the space increases four or five-fold. There must also be a gap of a metre or two to allow for safety margins. This may be another minor factor in the small number of people practising Tai Chi weapons today.

THE 13 POSTURE SWORD FORM

Below are some names given by Yearning K Chen to the 13 actions in the 13 Posture Sword Form:

Ch'ou – lashing	Peng – snapping
T'ai – striking	Chiao – stirring
T'i – raising	Ya – pressing
Ke – blocking	Pi – splitting
Chi – piercing	Chieh – intercepting
Tz'u – stabbing	IIsi – clearing
Tien – pointing	

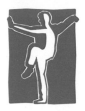

TAI CHI AND ALLIED MARTIAL ARTS

Whenever martial arts students and teachers get together, whatever their style or art, stories and gossip about martial arts are handed around, endless comparisons between techniques are made, arguments about the past rage in a friendly way, and occasionally someone will rise to his feet and demonstrate a point. In short, the bonhomie of 'insiders' the world over permeates the group. In such surroundings, you always hear about something that you did not know about before; about different arts, teachers and events. This was the same in the past, and may partly explain why students who have been devoted to one style for a long time sometimes leave it and go to learn another art.

TAI-KI-KEN

A modern, documented example of this is Kenichi Sawai, a Japanese man born in 1903. At the age of 22, he was already a 5th Dan Black Belt in Judo, a 4th Dan in Kendo and a 4th Dan in Laido, the art of drawing and using a real sword. When he was 28, he visited China, where he heard about a martial artist called Wang Hsiang-ch'i. Wang was a famous Hsing-I teacher of the Honan school. When Wang was proficient in Hsing-I, he changed the name of his art to I-Ch'uan (Mind Boxing).

After a short period of 'Knocking on the door', Kenichi Sawai managed to arrange a meeting with Wang, and the inevitable test of skills ensued. Sawai wrote: 'When I had my first opportunity to try myself in a match with Wang, I gripped his right hand and tried to use a technique. But I at once found myself being hurled through the air. Next I tried grappling. I gripped his left hand and his right lapel and tried the techniques I knew, thinking that, if the first attacks failed, I would be able to move into a grappling technique (fighting on the floor) when we fell. But the moment we came together, Wang instantaneously gained complete control of my hand and thrust it out and away from himself.' Kenichi Sawai was still not deterred and requested a contest with sticks, to stand in place of swords. The Japanese sword expert could not touch Wang. However, Wang accepted Sawai as a pupil.

Within the teaching of Hsing-I or I-Chu'uan was a branch known as Ta-ch'eng-ch'uan. Sawai studied this, and when he was competent in the art, Wang gave him permission to start teaching it in Japan. He renamed the art Tai-ki-ken, which is the Japanese rendering of Tai Chi Ch'uan although it does not resemble Tai Chi very much.

The foundation training for Wang's Hsing-I was standing meditation. This meditation method in a standing position is said to arouse very active modes of Chi, vital energy, and give students a kind of springing, animal power of movement.

There are five basic techniques of Hsing-I – splitting, crushing, drilling, pounding and crossing. In addition to these five techniques, there are 12 methods of moving based on the actions of animals; dragon, tiger, horse, monkey, cock, hawk, iguana, snake, eagle, bear, swallow and ostrich.

A low, crouching stance, reminiscent of the tiger movements, is adopted for many of the movements of Tai-ki-ken, reminding us of Tai Chi. Today, many exponents of Tai Chi stand high; that is, with only a slight knee bend and tucking in of the joints at the groin.

But if you look at old photographs of Yang Cheng-fu and Chen Wei-ming, you will see that they are low.

There is also a method of driving down an opponent's arms in Tai Chi Combat, which is very similar to some of the techniques of Tai-ki-ken. However, there is not the same softness in the action of Tai-ki-ken as there is in Tai Chi, and also Tai-ki-ken is completely geared towards fighting.

These two examples of martial artists with a mixed background bring into focus the question of the purity of an art such as Tai Chi. Wherever we look, we cannot find the 'pure' style or stylist. Whoever we examine, we find that either he or she, or their teaching itself has been influenced by another martial art or by another style of Tai Chi. Everyone is doing a variation on something else.

SUN LU-T'ANG

Sun Lu-t'ang, (see chapter 1) was a student and teacher of three arts: Tai Chi, Hsing-I and Pa-kua. His early training emphasizes that although Tai Chi is soft, the softness requires very hard training to acquire. Kuo Yun-shen was one of Sun's Hsing-I teachers. Kuo would mount a horse, make Sun hold on to the horse's tail, and ride for long distances with his pupil tagging on behind.

Sun's skill increased as he was trained, but one day he met his match. He heard a man coming up behind him to attack, and tried to seize the man. The assailant avoided his move and try as he might, Sun could not grip him. The stranger turned out to be a Taoist. He taught Sun how to cultivate his Chi and gave him dietary advice, including changing to a vegetarian diet.

Sun's powers also extended to healing, horse riding, fighting with a staff and archery.

PA-KUA CHANG

Yang style Tai Chi is the most popular form of Tai Chi outside Asia. It features very few clenched fist techniques. The chief formation of the hand found in the style is the open palm. This is also the chief hand formation in another internal art, Pa-kua Chang or Eight Trigram Boxing.

Though the origin of Pa-kua is not known, it is traditionally placed in the Ch'ing dynasty. Its documented history begins in the late 18th century with the appearance of a certain Wang Hsiang, from whom it was handed down to the present day. The techniques of the art include striking, seizing, tripping and throwing. It is known as a very fierce and powerful style. We in the West are not familiar with the use of the palm (heel) as a striking surface, as we regard the clenched fist as the most effective use of the hand as a weapon. However, the open palm is a very dangerous weapon when used by a trained practitioner. It has the advantage too of not being as dangerous to the user. It is much easier to injure the fingers and knuckles when the fist is clenched.

A striking feature of Pa-kua Chang is that students learn to 'walk the circle'. That is, the central method of training is to walk continuously in a circle, and then, following specific foot movements, to turn and retrace the same circle in the opposite direction. The open palms are held in such a way as to protect the head and trunk, and as the change in direction is made the hands twine around the body and back into their original position. This action of the hands is called Palm Changing, of which there are several variations of increasing complexity.

The use of the waist to effect turns, evasions and attacks is emphasized in Tai Chi traditional training, but in Pa-kua it is stressed even more. From a theoretical point of view the Eight Trigrams (*see* p.94), which were the basis of the 64 Hexagrams of the *I-Ching*, are mentally located at regular intervals around the circle that the Pa-kua student walks. Each Trigram is placed at a

69

particular point on the eight compass directions and has its own special meaning and qualities associated with it. The idea is that the student is mindful of these eight places as he walks the circle. If we take the *I-Ching*'s description of the Eight Trigrams, we have the attributes of Strong, Yielding, Inciting Movement, Dangerous, Resting, Penetrating, Light-giving, Joyful, and corresponding images of Heaven, Earth, Thunder, Water, Mountain, Wind, Fire, Lake. Picture the Pa-kua student as he moves round the circle, keeping his body relaxed and vertical, and imagining these different qualities as he passes their corresponding points. His leading hand is directed to the centre of the circle and his gaze follows his hand, to a place from which all this emanates. We have here all the hallmarks of some kind of ritual that is far removed from ideas of combat.

Since the Eight Trigrams were originally thought of as representations of all that happens in Heaven and on Earth, perhaps students of Pa-kua are meant to be immersing themselves in this representation as they move. In the main, however, this kind of mental process is not followed by Pa-kua enthusiasts in the Western world.

As in Tai Chi Combat, the fighting side of Pa-kua makes use of what we can call 'recoil' energy. For instance, if the waist is twisted to the left to send out the right palm, the recoil of the waist – the twist-back of the waist – sends out the left palm with even greater force. This is also true of the Japanese art of Aikido, which we shall come to later.

Pa-kua, Hsing-I and Tai Chi, then, are the Chinese trio of internal arts. They have all been connected with the Eight Trigrams in some way, they all place emphasis on the mind-body relationship, have Taoist connections, rely on Chi power to some extent and continue to attract and delight Western students. Of the three, only Tai Chi has become widespread. This is probably due to the long, slow, solo forms of the latter; something that is missing in the other two.

CHIN-NA

In the Chinese language the word 'Chin' means to grab hold of, or seize, and the word 'Na' means to control or keep hold of. Combined, the two words give us the name of another martial art that is not very well known outside the martial arts circles – Chin-na, the art of gripping and holding.

In Tai Chi, movements such as Pull, Needle at Sea Bottom and Step Back to Drive Monkey Away, can be interpreted as seizing or holding techniques when applied to a partner. Part of a Chin-na student's training is to understand the joints of the body; how they can be twisted and locked. Another part is the study of vital points of the body, and at a deeper level to be aware of the flow by the use of pressure. A third aspect is the study of medicinal herbal remedies. When carried to extremes, Chin-na is a gruesome, horror-movie martial art, which we do not want to dwell on in a book about Tai Chi!

Some Tai Chi clubs concentrate some of their training time on examining how the body of the partner can be temporarily immobilized so that an unbalancing push can be given. In common with Tai Chi, Chin-na uses large, medium and small circles for its joint locking techniques. The development of a powerful grip using variations of finger and thumb is also important; for instance gripping only with the index finger and thumb, index and middle finger and thumb, and so on. In this connection one is reminded of Chen-style master, Chen Fake, who 'practised with a wooden staff about 4m long and 15cm thick. He shook the heavy thing 300 times a day as a way to exercise his wrist strength.' (Cheng Man-Ching, *Master Cheng's 13 Chapters on T'ai Chi Ch'uan*). Once, when attacked by a man with a spear, Chen gripped the haft of the weapon, gave a slight twist and jabbed the spear back at the man sending him some four metres away. This type of technique is found in the syllabus of Chin-na. If a martial art is to be effective in fighting, it must take into account as many circumstances that might arise as possible. The study of Tai Chi Combat shows that methods akin to those of Chin-na are essential.

AIKIDO

Although Aikido is a Japanese martial art it should be dealt with in this book because in the eyes of many martial artists, especially Westerners, it has some relationship with Tai Chi. The founder of Ai-ki-do (meeting of the Spirit Way) was Morihei Uyeshiba (1883–1969). He was the son of an influential farmer, with samurai ancestors, and the Kumano district where he was born was a traditional centre of Japanese mysticism. In common with other famous martial artists, both before and after him, Uyeshiba was a sickly child. The boy studied the religious texts of Shingon Buddhism, believed fervently in the Shinto gods of the national Japanese faith, and showed an uncommon interest in all religious matters. By subjecting himself to a spartan way of life, which included a daily dousing in ice cold water, Uyeshiba improved his health. He spent some time living in Tokyo but preferred a more rural life and returned to his own village. He had begun to study Jujitsu and found it an absorbing subject. He married, joined the army and studied all manner of martial arts.

Uyeshiba's desire to build up his physical strength and resistance to pain was extraordinary. According to biographer John Stevens, Uyeshiba used to pound his skull 'against a stone slab a hundred times a day'. In addition to the demands he made on his body, Uyeshiba was equally tormented by spiritual matters. His early life consisted of an endless search for something that he could not define. After some years of this, Uyeshiba met the last of the old-time Japanese warriors, Sokaku Takeda. This was a man who feared nothing and no-one. After being 'deftly handled' by Sokaku in a challenge contest, Uyeshiba became his pupil.

The martial art that Sokaku taught was called Daito Ryu. After a period of study, Uyeshiba once more went his own way. Sokaku, though a fighter without peer, did not have the character to match it, nor the thirst for spiritual fulfilment that Uyeshiba desired.

Uyeshiba's life story makes enthralling reading and what emerges from it is that he was a man susceptible to visions, capable of very unusual feats, apparently able to read the thoughts of those around him, and possessed of exceptional, irrepressible physical strength and energy. He once had a contest with an accomplished swordsman, an unarmed man against an armed one, and made it impossible for the attacker to strike him. Asked for an explanation of this he replied, 'Just prior to your attacks, a beam of light flashed before my eyes, revealing the intended direction.'

Although he lived in the 20th century, Uyeshiba's life reminds one of the ancient Taoist hermits who pepper the history of Chinese martial arts, performing their seeming miracles, overcoming all attacks and able to move with such speed that they virtually fly. Behind these external accomplishments hovers an invisible wisdom that makes everything possible. In common with Tai Chi masters of the past, Uyeshiba's training was physically severe (again, softness is built on strength). Aikido is an evasive, defensive, soft art compared with Karate or Jujitsu; whether the severe training is essential to such arts or simply commonly found is hard to say. Another interesting point of comparison between Uyeshiba and the Chen family members is that they all came from rural, farming backgrounds. This proximity to nature, in which most Taoist teachings are set, may be important.

In my view the two aspects of Aikido that are closest to the art of Tai Chi are the evasive footwork and body shifting, plus the use of the palms for pushing. The arm bending and locking of Aikido as an immediate counter-measure I have no time for, because the arms of a fighting man or woman cannot be bent and locked unless he is in such pain or a state of semi-consciousness or drunkenness that he cannot control them; or unless his physical strength is vastly inferior to that of his opponent. Perhaps Uyeshiba could have done these things. In the foot work and body shifting of Aikido through movement after movement there is an echo of the same sweeping and swirling, rising and falling energy that is found in the internal martial arts of China. When moving in this way, one experiences a kind of joy and exhilaration of movement.

THE ALEXANDER TECHNIQUE AND TAI CHI

Frederick Matthias Alexander, the founder of the Alexander Technique, was born in 1869. Alexander's early career involved speaking on stage, and he developed his system of posture and movement enhancement in response to a problem with his voice.

Alexander devised many methods, some of them involving the use of mirrors, to find out if, when he was speaking, he did something with his posture that interfered with the production of sound. After much research, he came to the conclusion that no matter how much effort he put into correcting his posture, he could not succeed. If he told himself to move a couple of centimetres this way or that way, or pull back his shoulders or raise his head, it made no difference. Habit, tension and, especially, wrongly interpreted sensations of his posture, always overcame his intentions. He realized that almost everyone's image of how he or she is standing or moving is in fact wrong. Alexander came to the conclusion that most of us need re-educating in terms of the way we use or bodies.

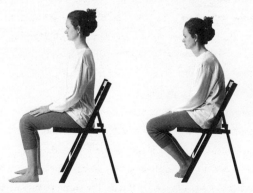

ABOVE THE ALEXANDER TECHNIQUE IS A FORM OF BODY RE-EDUCATION. PUPILS ARE TAUGHT HOW TO SIT AND STAND CORRECTLY, SO THAT THE HEAD, NECK AND SPINE ARE USED IN A NATURAL WAY.

The connection between the Alexander Technique and Tai Chi lies in several areas. One of the sayings of the Tai Chi classics is that the head should be suspended from above, as if held by a hair. For this to happen, the neck must be free, not fixed. This freeing of the neck is one of the main focuses of the Alexander system. In Tai Chi, the spine should be naturally erect and the centre of gravity lowered. For this to happen, the knees have to be slackened from their habitual tension and the sacral and lower lumbar vertebrae must be released from the unnecessary state of backward and upward pressure, caused by wrong muscular tension. This too is one of the results of Alexander training. Today it is not uncommon for Tai Chi and Alexander training to come together from time to time in special seminars.

TAI CHI AND FELDENKRAIS

Feldenkrais was interested in the relationship between posture and psychology. One of the subjects that interested him early in his career was the role of posture in sexual behaviour; that is, in making love. He found that many people with sexual problems were unable to move the pelvis freely backward and forward. The guilt they felt about sex and the sexual act more or less froze their pelvis on to their upper body.

Feldenkrais also had a black belt in Judo. When performing Judo, especially in fighting on the floor, the hips, waist and general pelvic area come in for a lot of movement. In Judo groundwork, the lower back must be flexible and free moving for a player to be successful. A Judoka (Judo student) with the same problems as the people with sexual problems would not be able to perform techniques successfully.

Similar things can be said about Tai Chi performance. Waist turning, rippling the waist and pelvis or making the pelvis undulate when pushing, are all examples of this. Freedom of the scapula or shoulder blade, to which about a dozen muscles are attached, is another example of the crossing of Tai Chi and Feldenkrais paths.

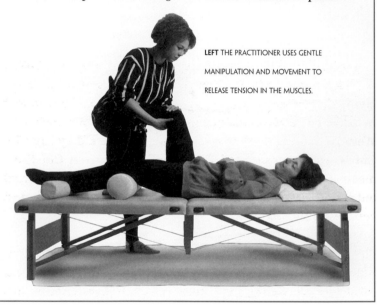

LEFT THE PRACTITIONER USES GENTLE MANIPULATION AND MOVEMENT TO RELEASE TENSION IN THE MUSCLES.

76

The subjects broached in this chapter, and many others, are clearly akin to Tai Chi in their several ways. This is because they all contain some kind of fundamental knowledge about the way we work, particularly with regard to how we move. Studying any one of them can throw light on the others and therefore increase our knowledge of ourselves.

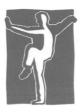

CHI KUNG

CHAPTER SIX

According to Greek mythology, there is a substance called *ichor*, which flows through the blood vessels of the gods, giving their blood a special quality. The Chinese believe that in addition to the energies in the human body detected by Western science, there is another energy, which they call Chi. Chi is usually translated as internal energy, and Chi Kung means the cultivation of internal energy. Chi Kung is carried out by adopting certain postures, regulating the breath and concentrating the mind.

Chi Kung extends back beyond the origins of Tai Chi forms. Authorities claim that the practice of Chi Kung can be traced back 4,000 years. The *Spring and Autumn Annals*, which are about 2,300 years old, state that people who live in damp, humid conditions, which lead to stagnation of the blood and spirits, are advised to do certain breathing exercises and to perform a kind of dance.

CHI

Chi can be thought of as a fine energy that assists and accompanies all the scientifically proven activities of the body and mind – breathing, digesting, seeing, homeostasis, thinking, feeling, moving, sensing, and so on. Anything that human beings do is assisted at some stage by Chi.

The influence of Chi Kung can be found in several fields, many of which affected the teaching and development of Tai Chi. Tai Chi students may find that it is useful to know something about these other influences so that when they meet them they will be able to identify their origin and assess how seriously or otherwise they want to take them.

MARTIAL ARTS

If we take styles of fighting that we are familiar with in the West, such as boxing, wrestling and even the Sumo tournaments that have become popular in recent years, we recognize the obvious fact that certain contestants have a clear superiority over the rest. Former heavyweight boxers Mike Tyson and Mohammed Ali are good examples. Chinese martial artists would say that the Chi of these two men was high, in the particular skill they had chosen. Theirs is hard Chi, and the Chi Kung they have, so to speak, unwittingly followed is Hard Chi Kung. Hard Chi is Chi that has been concentrated in the muscles to give extra power. Soft Chi is the Chi used in Tai Chi, Pa-kua and their offshoots, to increase sensitivity, lightness, agility and also power, but in a form different to the power of Hard Chi.

MEDICINE

The chief medical recognition of Chi lies in the application of fine needles to the acupuncture points, the burning of moxa powder on the same points, massage along the Chi channels and the palpation of the wrist pulses to ascertain the quality of Chi in various organs. It also concerns the yin and yang qualities of foods and herbs that affect the Chi and the use of medically supervised Chi Kung exercises.

One of the chief causes of illness, according to traditional Chinese medicine, is stagnant Chi, or stasis. For instance, a case of poor blood

RIGHT MOXA POWDER CAN BE APPLIED TO THE END OF AN
ACUPUNCTURE NEEDLE, AS HERE, OR DIRECTLY TO THE SKIN.
THE WARMTH STIMULATES STAGNANT CHI.

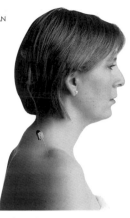

circulation might be diagnosed as connected with weak Chi of the blood, causing a slowing down of its movement and failure to penetrate fully into all the tiny blood vessels. On a mental level, we might say that stagnant Chi contributes to the syndrome of continually worrying about the same problem – mental stasis.

Chi Kung therapy helps many complaints, including gastric and duodenal ulcers, headaches, poor eyesight, stomach ache, neurasthenia and spastic colon. Chi Kung therapy stimulates and balances the flow of Chi, allowing the body to return to good health.

Chi Kung therapy is divided into two parts – static and dynamic. In static Chi Kung, a number of different postures are adopted; standing still, leaning, sitting, squatting, lying back and lying down. In the dynamic therapy, different postures, one after the other, are carried out. Some of them are designed to improve the general health and others are aimed at specific ailments.

79

THE FROLICS OF THE FIVE ANIMALS

The famous 2nd century Chinese doctor, Hua Tuo, wrote that the hinge on a door that is often used will never become covered with insects or infected by them, meaning that exercise and stretching helps to keep the body healthy.

He is credited with the invention of a series of movements. These movements, combined with breathing, were based on the 'frolics' of the Five Animals – bear, crane, deer, tiger and monkey. When a student performs these movements, their bearing and general demeanour should replicate not only the movements but also the spirit and feelings of the animal concerned.

The characteristics of the Frolics are:
- Mind and body working together.
- Flexible, spiralling and circular movements.
- Slow movements and fast movements.
  Slow 'like spinning silk' and fast 'like a frightened snake'.
- Appreciation of weight, stability and subtlety.
- Softness and hardness to appear according to the
  type of movement.
- Breathing to be in harmony with movement.
- Persevering and conscientious practice.

When the Frolics are performed, the student tries to see inside the animal and catch its spirit. For instance, although the bear is heavy and lumbering, it is nevertheless quick and agile when necessary. The crane flies as if it were 'playing with clouds and the moon', yet also stands 'as tranquil as a pine tree'. The deer leaps and darts, but is also very relaxed. The tiger has powerful claws and its eyes are filled with power; its movements 'suggest a hurricane' but also 'contain the quietude of the moon'. The monkey, though playful and constantly busy, nevertheless has its own kind of stillness.

The Five Frolics, therefore, are much more varied and versatile than the type of Tai Chi we generally see in the West. Their moods change markedly compared with the mood of Tai Chi, which emphasizes stillness and a kind of slow and measured dignity. However, when we come to some of the older forms of Tai Chi and their application to combat, we find closer links with the Five Frolics.

MASSAGE

The other aspect of Chi Kung therapy that is sometimes taught in Tai Chi classes is self-massage. We have all knocked an elbow or knee and instinctively placed a hand on it. This is partly to touch the spot and find out what has happened, but we also 'believe', without putting it into words, that we will 'make it better'. Mothers comfort fallen children with their hands. This widespread belief in the healing power of the hands has been extended in some detail in Chi Kung therapy. Techniques include patting with the palm, tapping with the tips of the fingers, stroking with the palm, twisting, poking, pressing, kneading, pinching, rubbing, chopping, seizing and pounding. In some cases, chop sticks, bamboo and padded sticks are applied instead of the hands. In fact, the actions are very similar to the hitting methods of martial arts; just the manner of using the hand and the intention are different.

The chief difference between Western massage and Chi Kung massage, sometimes called acupressure, is in the detailed focus of the hand and the theory behind it. In addition, acupressure uses stroking and tapping movements along the Chi channels of the body. In some Tai Chi classes these types of movement are taught for self-administration, to loosen up the body, dispel tension and try to bring the centre of gravity down, clearing the thoughts.

THE ARTS

By cultivating the Chi, mainly through the use of breath, painters, musicians, actors and calligraphers have been able to produce works and skills that are said to be impossible without the Chi.

The beauty of Chinese dancing is due in part to the use of Chi Kung. There is a chapter devoted to ancient music in the *Spring and*

Autumn Annals. This work tells how dances were devised to increase the fitness of the people.

Chang Chung-yan, in his book *Creativity and Taoism*, wrote: 'We find that the great masters of painting make their contributions only when they ... dwell in a state of inner serenity.'

This idea of inner serenity and the release of potentialities through the brush, of being in harmony with movement, yang, and quiescence, yin, are part and parcel of the gentle use of Chi, harmonizing with Chi. They are also to be found in Tai Chi forms.

Tai Chi is sometimes called meditation in movement, but it could equally be called painting in movement, since both the painter and student of the form rely on similar factors. The movement of Tai Chi is carried out against a background of inner stillness. Similarly, the movement and life of a Chinese painting owes much to the presence of a stillness in the open spaces of the painting contrasting with the action of a figure or wind-swept tree, or a 'rooted' mountain contrasting with the motion of a bird in flight.

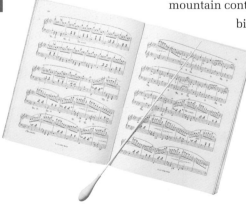

LEFT MUSICIANS RELY ON THEIR CHI TO HELP PRODUCE INNOVATIVE AND BEAUTIFUL MUSICAL SCORES.

TAOISM

From the point of view of Taoist philosophy, a person who tries to follow the Taoist Way is one who tries to understand and harmonize with natural energies through movement and stillness.

Harking back to the Zen abbot Takuan, and the letter he wrote to Yagyu about swordsmanship, we find a kind of Chi Kung that is more akin to that of the Chinese painters. He was speaking about the mind's tendency to 'stop' or stick to what it perceived. Later he enlarges his theme and says:

'When I look at a tree, I perceive one of its leaves is red, and my mind 'stops' with this leaf. When this happens, I see just one leaf and fail to take cognizance of the innumerable other leaves of the tree ... But when the mind moves on without 'stopping', it takes up hundreds of thousands of leaves without fail. When this is understood we are Kwannons (enlightened beings).'

The Chi Kung at work here is subtle, requiring hard work, preparation and long study. For Tai Chi students, it gives a picture of the uninterrupted doing of the forms or Push Hands with a perfect balance between movement and stillness. Takuan goes on to say that once the swordsman has become fully matured in the doctrine of no-mindedness (no-mind-stopping-ness), he is in a sense just as innocent of sword technique as he was before he ever saw or heard of a sword. Yet now, of course, he has changed.

By pursuing the aim of no-mind under the guidance of a teacher, a student is refining his Chi, is doing Chi Kung. It is enough to search repeatedly for relaxation and inner centring, which will lead to no-mind. It is not necessary to clutter up the mind with literally hundreds of theories and practices connected with the Taoist religion, especially when they are learned from books; this leads to everything-in-the-mind, not no-mind.

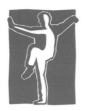

THE I-CHING, YIN-YANG AND THE FIVE ELEMENTS

CHAPTER SEVEN

The first part of this chapter will deal with the history and development of the *I-Ching*, the yin-yang concept and the five element theory. Their relationship with Tai Chi will be discussed in the second part of the chapter.

THE *I-CHING*

According to one Chinese tradition, the basis for the book that we know as the *I-Ching* or Book of Changes, was laid down by Fu Hsi (2852–2738 BC), the first legendary ruler of China. Others, however, maintain that the *I-Ching* was invented by King Wen (1184–1135 BC). The more modern scholars adhere to the theory that neither Fu Hsi nor King Wen had anything to do with it. This latter theory points out that during the Shang dynasty (1766–1123 BC), there was a method of divination that 'consisted of

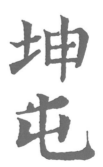

ABOVE THE CHINESE CHARACTERS FOR THE I CHING, OR THE BOOK OF CHANGES.

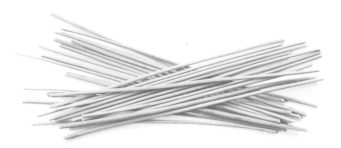

ABOVE YARROW STALKS ARE COMMONLY USED IN *I-CHING* DIVINATION. TRADITIONALLY, 49 STICKS ARE USED DURING AN *I-CHING* CONSULTATION.

applying heat to a shell or bone until cracks appeared. The form of the cracks determined the answer to the subject of divination'.

During this period, tribes of Tibetan and Turkish immigrants moved into the present Shensi province and founded the Chou state. The worship of the heavens, stars and sun was prominent in their religion, and may have contributed to the hierarchical view of the universe that is found in the *I-Ching*. In 1122 BC, the Chou dynasty replaced the Shang and lasted until 249 BC. It is said that during the Chou dynasty steps were taken to make the traditional divination process clearer. It is believed that during the early Chou the oracle bones were set aside in favour of a method using yarrow stalks. A fixed number of stalks were used in a certain order and yielded various combinations so that a codified series of interpretations could be drawn up.

Scholars believe that the yarrow stalks were the basis for the lines of the *I-Ching*. At its outset the book was a collection of linear signs. There were only two types of line. One was an unbroken straight line, and the other a line of equal length, divided into two equal parts. At first the lines were arranged in groups of three, one line on top of the other, in different series, to give the Eight Trigrams. Depending on which series emerged during the process of divination, the *I-Ching* could be consulted and the verdict given. Once again, there is no information about the earliest development of this method. We can only assume that from the early interpretations some of them became the accepted and traditional ones and the rest were discarded.

Gradually, a picture emerges of a book that grew and spread, both in content and influence. It is said that Confucius (551–479 BC) expressed the wish that if he could live for another 100 years he would like to spend 50 of them studying the *I-Ching*.

During the later part of the Chou dynasty, but before the time of Confucius, the official Eight Trigrams were combined into groups of 6 lines, to give 64 hexagrams and interpretations.

Later, appendices called the Ten Wings were added to the *I-Ching*. It is only in the Ten Wings that we find references to yin and yang. It seems that the introduction of yin-yang theory as such into *I-Ching* interpretation was a later event. Prior to it, the yin-yang school of thought apparently existed separately.

From the early centuries of the Christian period up to the present time, a multitude of interpretations and uses of the *I-Ching* have been made. The power and vagueness of the book attracts, confuses, enlightens and delights its devotees. Because the yin-yang concept is shared also by the Taoist religion and philosophy, all three streams, originally quite separate, of *I-Ching*, yin-yang and Taoism, have appeared in Tai Chi theory. Before leaving the *I-Ching* for a moment we should see some of the trigrams and hexagrams, together with examples of their interpretation.

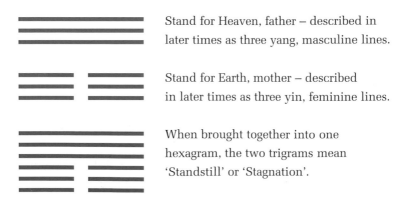

Stand for Heaven, father – described in later times as three yang, masculine lines.

Stand for Earth, mother – described in later times as three yin, feminine lines.

When brought together into one hexagram, the two trigrams mean 'Standstill' or 'Stagnation'.

A hexagram can be seen from one point of view as consisting of two trigrams, one on top of the other. According to I K Shchutskii in his book, *Researches on the I-Ching*:

'In the theory of the Book of Changes, the lower trigram is customarily regarded as referring to the internal life, to what is coming, to what is being created, and the upper trigram to the external world, to what is receding, to what is dissolving.'

In the hexagram for Standstill shown above, the yang is diminishing and the yin is increasing. Leaving aside the traditional interpretations of the *I-Ching* we could see this hexagram of two trigrams as a picture of the increasing role of women in our society and the diminishing role of men!

Finally, the lines were each given a number, starting from the bottom line, from one to six. For divinatory purposes, different attributes were allocated to each line. One such, quoted by Shchutskii, is as follows:

87

Line 6 represents the Head
Line 5 the Shoulders
Line 4 the Torso
Line 3 the Thighs
Line 2 the Shins
Line 1 the Feet

If taken in a completely literal sense, such an equation of parts of the body with the lines of the hexagrams could be the basis of a relationship between the *I-Ching* and a complete system of martial arts.

Let's leave the last word in this section to Joseph Needham, the world famous authority on Chinese history and culture:

*'The key word in Chinese thought is Order and above all
Pattern. Things behave in particular ways not necessarily
because of prior action or impulsions of other things, but
because their positions in the ever-moving cyclical universe
was such that they were endowed with intrinsic natures
which made that behaviour inevitable for them.'*

The changing picture presented by the 64 hexagrams is an ideal
expression of the above. The position of a line in the hexagram
determines its pathway or direction; its intrinsic nature, broken or
unbroken, makes its behaviour inevitable and its relationship with the
other lines modifies both its direction and the expression of its nature.

YIN-YANG

The yin-yang concept was developed by early Chinese cosmologists.
Their thinking gave rise to the Yin-Yang Chia or Yin-Yang school. The
word yin originally referred to the dark side of a hill or mountain,
where the sun did not reach, and the word yang to the light side,
illuminated by the sun.

It is not known when these terms were first used in connection
with Chinese explanations of the origin and growth of the universe.
According to the classification of Chinese schools made by Ssu-ma
T'an in the 2nd century BC, the Yin-Yang Chia was separate from the
Tao-Te Chia or School of the Way and its Power, which was the early
school of Taoist philosophy. During the Han dynasty, before the
Christian era, the yin-yang concept attracted a great deal of attention.
People using the *I-Ching* for divination found in the two words some
new inspiration.

The meaning of the two words gradually widened from that of
two primal creative forces to mean such things as: yin — cold,
rest, responsiveness, passivity, darkness, interiority, downwardness,
inwardness and decrease; and yang — heat, stimulation, movement,

activity, excitement, vigour, light, exteriority, upwardness, outwardness and increase. The yin-yang concept and the *I-Ching* exerted a reciprocal action on one another's interpretation.

Since, to state the obvious, we distinguish between things by observing their distinctions and assemble things by observing their similarities, the concept of yin and yang can be an amazingly useful tool for analyzing many types of activity. However, it is important to

YIN-YANG AND THE BODY

The concept of yin-yang has an empirical basis in Chinese traditional medicine, where it has been tested for centuries. A high fever represents a yang condition, and a state of cold shock a yin condition.

The organs of the body are classified into the two divisions and treated accordingly.

Yin	Yang
Heart	Small Intestine
Lungs	Large Intestine
Pericardium	Stomach
Spleen	Gall Bladder
Liver	Bladder
Kidneys	Triple Burner
	(not an organ in itself but a
	relationship between organs)

The most famous Chinese medical treatise is the *Nei Ching Su Wen*, known in English as *The Yellow Emperor's Book of Internal Medicine*. It is first mentioned in the *Annals of the Former Han Dynasty*, (206 BC–AD 25). The yin-yang concept, the Five Element theory and the concept of Chi all appear within this book.

bear in mind that they do not describe fixed states. Both are continually changing because of the action of the one upon the other, or rather because the activity of the one evokes the activity of the other. The appeal of such a concept to the Taoists was strengthened by the fact that Taoism has no explicit idea of a Creator. Their interest lies in order and patterns of events. The universe can be seen as a gigantic interplay of yin and yang. Within each yin there is some yang to be found and within each yang some yin.

The diagram used by the Chinese to express the yin-yang concept is shown on p.47. It is the diagram of the 'two fishes', one white and one black with 'eyes' of the opposite colour. Black stands for yin and white for yang. The eyes indicate that in the phenomenal world neither aspect exists in its pure form but always contains something of its opposite.

THE FIVE ELEMENTS

The Chinese word *Hsing* means to act or to do. *Wu* is the word for five, and so *Wu Hsing* means the Five Activities, the Five Things That Are Being Done. The expression is found in *Shou Ching*, the *Book of History*, compiled by Confucius. Though traditionally given a date or origin some 2,000 years BC by those who wished to confer the respectability of great age upon it, modern scholarship places the Wu Hsing theory some time in the third or fourth centuries BC.

In the early stages, the Wu Hsing theory involved thinking in terms of the actual substances, water, fire, metal, etc. Later on, their meaning became more abstract. The Wu Hsing was developed by the Yin-Yang Chia in the thinking about 'the mutual influence between nature and man' and represents a simple scientific attempt to explain the universe's activity. It was a later phase of the Yin-Yang Chia that stated that the interaction of yin and yang produces the Five Activities.

In most English translations of the expression Wu Hsing, the word 'element' has been chosen in preference to 'activity'. This may have been because we have the idea of Four Elements in our own culture. Such a facile translation has led to a lot of misunderstanding because our conception of an element, from school days, is of a substance that, until the coming of atomic fission, could not be broken down into smaller parts. This is the very antithesis of the later use of the Wu Hsing, both in its philosophical and medical applications. The Five Activities of Water, Fire, Wood, Metal, Soil (Earth) are processes, in movement, and they interact. For instance, Water puts out Fire, Fire burns Wood, and so on.

Apart from this literal relationship, any activity that can be equated with Water, or placed in the same category as Water, tends to quell any Fiery type of activity. This is important because we in the West tend to look for cause and effect; action number one produces result number two. The Five Activities do not so much cause something to happen as create a pattern in which something does happen. It is in their nature to be and act as they are.

When the number Five is applied to certain phenomena, it fits into it nicely, as for instance in the case of the four seasons. There are four seasons and the balance that exists between them makes up the

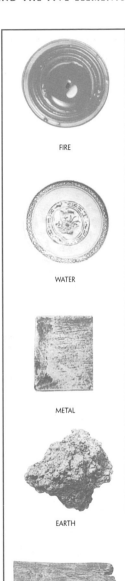

FIRE

WATER

METAL

EARTH

WOOD

91

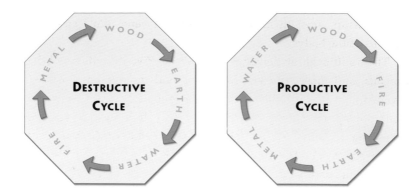

ABOVE THE FIVE ELEMENTS ARE LINKED INTO A NEVERENDING CYCLE OF PRODUCTIVE AND DESTRUCTIVE PROCESSES. IN THE PRODUCTIVE CYCLE, EACH ELEMENT CREATES THE NEXT IN THE CYCLE. IN THE DESTRUCTIVE CYCLE, EACH ELEMENT DESTROYS THE NEXT IN THE CYCLE.

number to five. Wood represents the state of things in growth, therefore springtime; Fire the state of things that has reached maximum phase, and so summer; Metal a declining state, autumn, and Water a state of rest, winter. Earth or Equilibrium is the natural balance between the four, the place where they intermingle but do not intrude upon one another.

The tendency to preserve and glorify the past, no matter what, led the proponents of the Wu Hsing into problems that can once more be illustrated by medicine. Below is a table showing the

	Wood	Fire	Earth	Metal	Water
Yin Organ	Liver	Heart	Spleen	Lungs	Kidneys
Yang Organ	Gall Bladder	Small Intestine	Stomach	Large Intestine	Bladder

relationship given in medicine to yin and yang, Wu Hsing and organs of the body.

The traditional relationships between the Five Activities and the organs, and those between the organs and the yin-yang concept were frequently at odds with one another. The Five Activities interpretation could say that the 'liver opens into the eyes' and the yin-yang that the 'Chi of all organs is reflected in the eyes' (T Kaptchuk, *The Web that has no Weaver*).

Kaptchuk continues by saying:

> *'Five Phases (Activities) theory emphasizes one to one correspondences, while yin-yang theory emphasizes the need to understand the overall configuration upon which the part depends ... The Five Phases became a rigid system ... yin-yang theory ... with its emphasis on a Taoistic view of the importance of the whole, allowed for a great deal of flexibility.'*

93

An interesting footnote as far as Tai Chi students are concerned, is that neither Lao-tzu nor Chuang-tzu refer to the Five Activities, Phases or Elements, but they do refer to yin-yang theory. As quotations from both these sage sources are often cited by Tai Chi writers and teachers, this is significant.

This rigidity of the Five Activities theory has caused a lot of 'fudging' by the medical practitioners who have been determined to make it work in every case. From the moment the theory was written down, it was criticized.

Kaptchuk gives the view that the Five Activities became 'entrenched' in the thinking of Chinese medicine because 'Chinese investigative study tends to be inductive only to a point and then proceeds with deductions based on the classics ... Most modern Chinese critics describe Five Phases theory as a rigid metaphysical overlay on the practical and flexible observations of Chinese medicine.' This is reflected in the attitude of martial arts theorists.

The original name of Hsing-I Ch'uan could well have been Five Activities Boxing, since its basic movements consist of five techniques. Pa-kua took its name from the Eight Trigrams and Tai Chi from the diagram of the Supreme Ultimate. Tai Chi theory also takes the Eight Trigrams and relates them to eight movements or gates and subdivided these into four directions and four corners.

	Ward Off	Sky	South
	Roll-Back	Earth	North
	Press	Water	West
	Push	Fire	East
	Elbow	Lake	Southeast
	Split	Thunder	Northeast
	Pull	Wind	Southwest
	Shoulder	Mountain	Northwest

The relationship of these movements to the directions and corners makes no sense at all from a logical point of view. The first four movements in the list of eight are all performed in roughly the same direction in forms. The eight movements do not have any logical relationship either with the meanings of the trigrams nor of the phenomena associated with them. The two exceptions are Ward Off and Roll-Back, Sky (Heaven) and Earth. Here the three Yang lines denote strong action, which does relate to Ward Off, and the three weak lines of Roll-Back's trigram, Earth, denote yielding action. Attempts have been made to justify the six remaining movements with the meanings of the trigrams, but they are very weak. For instance, it has been said the movement Press is like water, because water gradually wears away the hardest stone by dripping. The movement of Push, Fire, has been described as very aggressive, like fire burning through a forest. But both of these things can be said about both of the movements willy-nilly, with the kind of associative arguments that are used by students in their appreciations of literature.

Other writers and teachers have taken this process even further and tried to relate Tai Chi to the hexagrams. If the process of relating movements to the trigrams was subjective and fanciful, then that of relating them to the hexagram is even more so. A Tai Chi student may, over a long period, develop his or her own personal affinity with the *I-Ching* and connect its hexagrams with thoughts and feelings, imagination and sensations, but in my view this does not constitute a real, objective relationship at all.

Two versions of an interpretation of one of the hexagrams follows. Both will be seen to be valid. The process can be compared with a woman who goes to see a fortune teller. The fortune teller says that the woman is going to have news that will please her, but she may not recognize it as good news at first; that she must be alert also to her financial situation because if she is not she may run into difficulties; that there is a man she knows who thinks highly of her but something in her character is stopping him from saying so. These things said are so general that they could be said with equal validity to any normal person, man or woman. They can be interpreted in dozens of ways, all equally possible. They do not represent telling the future at all. Similarly, the generalized meanings of the *I-Ching* cannot be applied to specific movements exclusively in any way that satisfies me, and I started off as someone who was quite happy to be a believer.

The hexagrams are approached in divination by dividing the six lines into two trigrams. This is the main and obvious division. Lines four, five, six make up the upper trigram and lines one, two, three the lower. Within the hexagram there are two that are called nuclear trigrams; the word nuclear having been chosen presumably because they lie inside, like a nucleus. The nuclear trigrams are taken from lines two, three, four, five and overlap one another. Lines two, three, four make up the lower trigram and lines three, four, five the upper. This means that lines three and four are common to both though they have different places in each.

Having clarified for oneself the type of trigram according to the above method, the first step is to look at what is called the Time. The category of Time gives the overall meaning of the hexagram: does it show increase or decrease? does it assist a process or cause conflict? how long will it last? and so on. The next category is called Place. This consists of examining each line, registering its position and its significance with regard to the other lines. There are other considerations, but this is enough to show that the interpretation of a hexagram is a complex subject. According to Richard Wilhelm:

> *'Since the Han period... more and more mystery and finally more and more hocus-pocus have become attached to the book. Though I may be shot down in flames for saying so I find that attempts to relate the hexagrams to Tai Chi movements does verge on "hocus-pocus"'.*

INTERPRETING THE HEXAGRAM

1. If we place the hexagram Ch'ien in front of a person performing the Tai Chi movement Ward Off Left and Ward Off Right in such a way that it is evenly spread, the fifth line is level with his jaw. When the left hand rises in Ward Off Left it reaches the level of the jaw, the fifth line. The existence of six strong lines in this

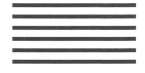

ABOVE THE CH'IEN OR CREATIVE HEXAGRAM IS MADE UP OF SIX UNBROKEN LINES.

hexagram evokes an image of strength and awakening, indeed of the stirring dragons mentioned in the *I-Ching's* interpretation of it. The second line's interpretation speaks of a 'dragon appearing in the field'. The field can represent the abdomen. If, in the next movement of Ward Off Right, the rising hand goes too far, above the chin or fifth line, and reaches the sixth line, then according to the *I-Ching* an 'arrogant dragon will have cause to repent', meaning that the movement will look ugly and awkward.

This interpretation takes as its basis the position of the lines and the position of the hands in the movements concerned. In the case of the fifth line the hand position rising to the jaw is taken in a spatial sense, and the case of the second line is taken in a different sense altogether, because the second line is not level with the abdomen, but much further down. The idea of 'field' is found in some translations as the Tan T'ien, a point just below the navel, which is given in English as 'cinnabar field'. It can also mean Earth.

2. If we take once more as our example the *I-Ching's* interpretation of the first line, which is 'hidden dragon, do not act' and say that this means that the lower legs and feet are filled with hidden power, ready to move when the time is right. The second line, 'dragon appearing in the field', means that the hidden power is projected into the whole body, or we could say into the Tan T'ien, cinnabar field, like celestial forces appearing on Earth (field). The left hand rises like

97

a dragon in the sky and the right hand settles down, towards the Earth. This means that although the energy rises, it is also at the same time rooted. One must beware of raising the left hand too high, to the sixth line, because this is the place of the 'arrogant dragon' and an arrogant dragon opens itself to attack. The sixth line, being a yang line at the end of a series of five yang lines, means that activity has reached its maximum and the only possibility is now to yield, return to yin.

With a little imagination and ingenuity, combined with the right vocabulary, anyone can wander through the 64 hexagrams and produce highly plausible interpretations for all of them. Taking only the basic 13 postures and the 64 hexagrams, this would give us a total of a minimum of 832. If one then began to incorporate two, three or four hexagrams together then the number could rise to astronomic figures. At its best it seems that the *I-Ching* is a stimulus to thought and reflection about the possible movement inherent in Tai Chi, but direct and definitive interpretations are highly questionable.

It is in the application of yin-yang theory that Tai Chi finds its most helpful philosophical ally. As we saw in the chapter on postures, we can give every posture-movement a predominantly yin or yang label. Advancing or retreating, shifting weight from one leg to the other making one leg full and the other one empty, can all be seen from a yin-yang standpoint. This is, however, only a superficial and obvious analysis. For instance in the movement of Roll-Back, student A pushes student B. In doing Roll-Back, B rests the inside of his right forearm on the outside of A's pushing left arm. B withdraws his body, retreating, yin and diverts the push. Though B is retreating and yielding and so can be placed in the yin category, he is also diverting so using a little yang force. But as the yang force of the diverting action is also making use of the yin force of the whole retreating body it contains some yang force. Furthermore, because B does not so to speak fly back or fall back like a stone in a vacuum, we can say that his overall yielding body action is supported by yang acting as a brake, modifying the chief yin movement.

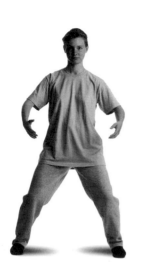
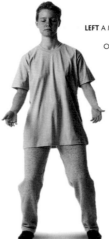

LEFT A MOVEMENT OR POSTURE IS YIN OR YANG DEPENDING ON HOW YOU PERFORM IT.

By painstakingly analysing the directions and actions of B's body, we find a whole network of yin and yang forces of varying degrees of strength all contained within the yin of his Roll-Back. In order for this analysis to be valid, the movements themselves must be correctly performed, in a relaxed state, and with every muscle producing just the amount of energy needed. If, for instance, the shoulders and arms are unnecessarily tense and the legs not firm, then the analysis that one could make for the ideal movement would no longer be valid.

Following in the footsteps of many other students of the Wu Hsing, Five Activities, Tai Chi practitioners have not been slow to find relationships. We looked earlier at the matter of difficulties that arose when this was done in the medical area and we find the same phenomenon in Tai Chi. One thesis that has been put forward is that there is a connection with five major organs of the body and five fundamental steps of the art: step forward, withdraw, look left, look right and balance. It is said that as each step is taken, the student is promoting the health of a specific organ. It hardly seems necessary to say that this kind of claim cannot be taken seriously. To criticize it further would be like hitting an unconscious opponent.

99

Similar efforts have been made rotating the Five Activities themselves in a circle and connecting them with the five steps: water puts out fire. Five words were chosen and called the Five Words Secrets. Par excellence, this demonstrates the taking of a revered idea from the past and fitting things in with it, no matter what the cost. As in the case of the *I-Ching*, endless arguments can be put forward to correlate the number five and Tai Chi. But the same can be achieved with three, four, six, seven, eight, nine as well. The idea of the Five Activities can be a stimulus and an intellectual basis for the Tai Chi beginner to start examining his movements. To try to fix oneself on that is a mistake.

What all three subjects of this chapter do is convey an idea of order and pattern to an art that is initially a difficult one for Westerners to appreciate. It is in this respect that they can be most useful. When one tries to relate the *I-Ching* and the Five Activities to Tai Chi in detail, then that detail is not a help but a stumbling block.

In my experience, the most important factor in developing one's Tai Chi is in exploring the meaning of relaxation. Relaxation means to increase one's sensitivity to the state of one's body. As this increases, then more and more unnecessary tensions are revealed. As they are revealed, they can be released. As they are released, then more subtle tensions are revealed, and so on. Relaxation leads to more relaxation, yin. And as the yin becomes clearer, then true, legitimate and necessary yang can be released at appropriate moments.

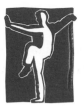

TAI CHI POETRY

CHAPTER EIGHT

A saying applied to the internal martial artist of China says, 'Looks like a Woman, Fights like a Tiger'. Training in the solo forms is certainly poetry in motion, and, equally, feminine on the outside but harbouring a tiger-like strength inside. When a student is able to do one of the forms in a satisfactory way, he or she experiences moods that can best be described as poetic, close to a religious experience.

There are a number of classic Tai Chi poems praising the art and reminding students of its fundamental direction, but the chief work outside these specifically Tai Chi poems is the *Tao Te Ching*. This book has inspired millions of people in as many ways.

One of the telling verses of the Tao Te Ching begins:

> *'There is no single thing in all the world softer than water, more supple than water; yet in all the world is there anything to equal water in overcoming things which are hard and strong.'*

This theme is repeated in a later verse with:

> *'When a man is born he is soft and supple, but when he dies he is stiff and hard. That which is stiff and hard belongs to death, but the soft and supple belong to life.'*

The *Tao Te Ching* asks us if we can become soft and supple, like a child, breathing like a child, being permeated by breath but not 'stopping' the mind at breathing. These inspiring words can help to evoke in a student a kind of 'right' feeling about what he or she is doing. The movement of the yang forms is continuous but should not become hard through the effort to be continuous. Students try to find a new rhythm in which continuity is not a strain, and breathing harmonizes with this rhythm. The muscles and joints of the body respond to this and enjoy it. It seems for a while as if one has become a human being.

Throughout the book there is a kind of spirit that cannot be defined; something that, like continuous movement, loses its essential quality as soon as one attempts to pin it down; 'Tao follows the laws of its own nature.' To try to pin it down, define it, is to try to change its nature.

Among the Tai Chi classics is an anonymous *Song of the 13 Postures*:

'Keep the 13 Postures close; do not forget them.
When wishing to move, start from the waist.
Be sensitive to the changes, the slightest shift from full to empty.
Thus you let the Chi circulate like a flow through all your body,
without ceasing.

Invisible in the embrace of stillness lies motion;
And within motion stillness is concealed.
Search, therefore, for that stillness within motion.
If you can approach this, discoveries will be yours
when you meet your opponent.

Let every movement be filled with awareness and meaning.
If you can approach this, the effort of no effort will appear.
Never abandon your attention to your waist.
When the abdomen is light and free, the Chi will be aroused.

When the lowest vertebrae are upright,
then the Spirit will rise to the top of the head.

The whole body should be pliant and soft,
The head suspended as if from above by a single hair.
Remain awake, searching for the meaning of Tai Chi itself.
Whether the body bends or stretches, whether it opens or closes,

Let the natural way be your way.
At the beginning, students listen to the words of their teacher,
But with care and effort they learn to apply themselves,
And then skill develops of its own accord.
Who can tell me, what is the main principle of Tai Chi?

The awakened mind comes first and the body will follow.
Who can tell me, what is the meaning and
philosophy of Tai Chi?
Eternal youthfulness and a healthy long life, which mean
An ever present springtime.
Each and every word of this song is valuable
and important to you;
If you do not listen to its words, and follow,
you will surely sigh your life away.'

Another, shorter anonymous instructional poem summarizes the actions of Push Hands. It is simply called *The Song of Push Hands*:

'When you use the actions of
Ward Off, Roll-Back, Press and Push,
Let them always be filled with meaning.
When you move, remember that every part of the body
is helped by another part.
If you move like this, no opening will appear
To let your opponent in.

> *If your opponent should use even the force of*
> *One thousand pounds against you,*
> *You can deflect it with the force of four ounces.*
> *Lead your opponent into you; let him lose his own balance.*
> *Combine yielding and attacking in one moment.'*

The famous Wang Tsung-yueh wrote an idealist description of Tai Chi mastery that is in a sense poetic. It is like a celebration of perfection in the art. He says:

> *'At the slightest pressure from an opponent, yield,*
> *and as soon as he begins to retreat, stick to him ...*
> *Match the speed of an opponent's movements, by*
> *moving quickly when he does, and slowly when he*
> *does. Whatever they may be, the multitude of*
> *techniques are governed by the same principle ...*
> *Train with diligence and so move on to intrinsic*
> *energy and so move on to enlightenment ... Talent,*
> *intuition, things of this kind are not enough without*
> *long persevering effort. The brain should be clear and*
> *empty, and the Chi lowered to the Tan T'ien, with an*
> *upright, relaxed body. Any change in your balance*
> *should be hidden from your partner.*
>
> *If you are pushed on your left side, it should be*
> *empty; If you are pushed on your right side, it should*
> *be empty. Wherever and whenever your opponent*
> *pushes you, he should find emptiness. As he comes*
> *forwards, your opponent should feel that he has*
> *leagues to go; as he goes backwards, he should feel*
> *hemmed in. If a feather drifted down on to your body,*
> *you would be so sensitive that you would feel it.*
> *If a fly were to settle upon you, you would be*
> *set in motion.'*

Wu Yu-seong, who changed from Yang to Chen style Tai Chi, also wrote about the art, along somewhat similar lines to Wang Tsung-yueh, but also speaking about the internal energies of the art. He had some striking similes.

'Let your spirit be like a cat catching a mouse.
Let your manner be like a hawk stooping for a rabbit.
Let your stillness be that of a mountain.
Let your movement be that of a river.
Gathering together your Chi should be like drawing a bow.
Releasing your Chi should be like loosing an arrow.
Your mind is the general, your Chi the flag,
your waist the flagpole.
When Ching moves, it should be like
the reeling in of silk.'

Other writers have tried to capture the spirit of Tai Chi in words but it is to these early works that students have turned time and again for guidance and a taste of the Supreme Ultimate.

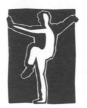

HERBAL REMEDIES AND FOOD

CHAPTER NINE

Wherever Chinese communities have been established, a herbal shop is sure to follow sooner or later. Rows and rows of carefully labelled boxes fill the shelves. On the counter are found clean sheets of paper piled up neatly beside a pair of scales. The customers file in, the assistants reach down the boxes, the contents are scooped out according to the prescription and wrapped up in the paper. Finally the contents of each packet are written in Chinese on the outside. This scene is, I guess, repeated the world over, because the Chinese people are great lovers of herbal remedies.

It is a tradition in Chinese martial arts circles that a full-time instructor studies healing to a certain extent, so that he can help his students in case of injury when training.

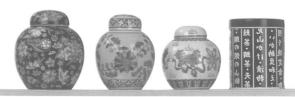

ABOVE CHINESE MEDICINE USES OVER 5,000 DIFFERENT HERBS AS WELL AS SOME MINERALS AND ANIMAL PARTS.

One of the commonest injuries is, of course, bruising. There is a common expression for the remedy for bruising – 'wine', so named because rice wine of good quality is used as a remedy base. Some 'wine' is drunk, to heal internal injuries and dissipate swelling, some 'wine' is applied to the bruise itself and some may be drunk and applied.

From the time of the Tang dynasty (618–907 AD) herbalism became the predominant Chinese medical approach. Today, there are far more Chinese physicians using herbs only to treat patients than there are ones using only acupuncture. The most recent pharmacopoeia lists 5,767 different herbs, minerals and animal extracts. It is important to distinguish between what we can call folk medicine and traditional medicine. Many of the popular beliefs about ginseng, for instance, belong in the folk category. Traditional herbalism classifies herbs according to their uses, not according to their chemical content. Herbs have a more specific and direct effect than acupuncture; the latter aims at the restoration of homeostasis rather than a specific cure. This means that herbs are more powerful and also can be more harmful if wrongly used. However, it seems that there are a series of traditional checks on the use of herbs that makes wrong prescription difficult.

If a student of Tai Chi is training in order to improve health, then some acquaintance with Chinese herbal knowledge may be a useful adjunct to this. At the same time, since the wrong use of herbs can be harmful, it is advisable to find a good, reputable herbalist and not rely on self-prescription.

The urino-genital system of the body has always been a focal point for some Tai Chi theorist. Though I guess that the majority of Chinese men and women make love in more or less the same passionate way as the majority of the rest of the world population and their intercourse goes through the same stages, there seems to have always been somewhere in the offing a different attitude, kept relatively secret in the past but appearing from time to time in published books. Part of this secret was the idea that if men and women could merely

GINSENG

The best known Eastern herb is of course ginseng, or *Panax Schinseng*, which belongs to the *Araliaceae* family. The word 'panax' comes from the same root as our 'panacea', meaning a cure for all things. Although, it is not used for any of the physical injuries caused by martial arts, it is high on the Chinese list of generally used herbs and has attracted a lot of attention in the West. It is a perennial herb and fetches a comparatively high price. Chinese herbalists insist that it will produce results such as increased metabolic rate, prevention of impotence, regulation of blood pressure and many other positive results.

Sir Edwin Arnold, the author of the book on the life of the Buddha, *The Light of Asia,* wrote of ginseng that 'it fills the heart with hilarity, whilst its occasional use will, it is said, add a decade to human life'.

LEFT GINSENG HAS BEEN USED IN THE EAST FOR THOUSANDS OF YEARS AS A TRADITIONAL CURE FOR IMPOTENCY AND GENERAL DEBILITY.

enjoy intercourse and not come to a climax on every occasion, they would enjoy better health and live longer. It is part of the tradition of some Chinese martial arts to refrain from intercourse when training is severe, so that the 'vital essence', the Ching or essence of sperm, should not be dissipated.

Whatever the wisdom of these ideas, and others like them, any method that could promote health in the kidneys, bladder and sexual organs was always treated with respect, whatever modern science might say about it now. A number of herbs were looked upon as aids in this search for such health.

Fo-ti-tieng is recommended in this respect, being good for the bladder. Juniper berries are used in teas, wines and oils for the kidneys and bladder, and since some types of back pain accompany disorders of the kidneys, juniper berries can also be said to be useful for relieving back pains. Other herbs for the kidneys and bladder are sage, marshmallow, divers and parsley piert.

One of the plagues of the male reproductive system is enlargement of the prostate gland, which presses on the urethra and prevents the passage of urine from the bladder. One of the herbs said to alleviate this complaint is parsley, prepared in the form of tea. The Chinese also recommend an extract of oats in fluid form to tone up the sexual organs, especially after over-indulgence. Ginseng appears once again, in this group of herbs, though it is not the aphrodisiac that it is sometimes claimed to be. The more sober Chinese users say that by slowly building up the general health through regular use, ginseng can restore sexual functioning to a better level.

MACROBIOTIC DIET

Over the last 20 years or so a new presentation of Eastern approaches to food and health has spread throughout the West in the form of the macrobiotic system. The chief promoter of macrobiotics has been the Japanese teacher, Michio Kushi. Though differing in many ways from traditional Chinese medical views, the basis of macrobiotics is said to be the ancient Yin-Yang Chia of philosophy. Since both the Chinese and macrobiotic systems are based on this ancient classification, the points on which they differ must be the result of a clash of interpretation. From its beginnings, macrobiotics centred on the understanding of food and drink and the classification of them into gradations of yin and yang. Then the sphere of its investigations extended into the worlds of exercise, acupressure, psychology and philosophy.

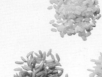

Here again the dangers of prescribing for oneself were evident when macrobiotics was a new craze, especially in the United States. Eating 'brown' or unpolished rice was one of the regular recommendations of macrobiotic specialists, as this particular food was seen as one which contained a balance of yin and yang qualities. Cases were reported of people putting themselves on a brown rice and water diet, and then suffering from malnutrition.

ABOVE RICE ALONE CANNOT PROVIDE A BALANCED DIET.

110

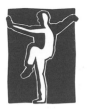

TAI CHI AND BREATHING

CHAPTER TEN

Early in 1990 I started a beginners' class in Tai Chi and after a few minutes I asked the class if there were any questions. One woman, a complete beginner, said, 'What about breathing?' This was a fair question because the subject of breathing does appear in books on Tai Chi. In reply I said what I always say – that if we learn the forms, do them in a relaxed way and at an even tempo, then the breathing will take care of itself. This is my attitude, because it is the most natural.

In the animal kingdom we find all kinds of movement and the movements of animals, birds, reptiles, fish and insects excel human movement in general. What animals have, and what we for the most part have lost, is the capacity not to interfere with our body movements. Tai Chi can be one of the things that helps us to undo that interference. To burden our bodies with breathing exercises on top of the mess we have already made of ourselves is to cause more problems.

An even more practical reason for leaving breathing exercises out of Tai Chi training, is that it is extremely difficult to learn the forms. If, as well as learning the forms, a student has to try to synchronize his breathing, control his abdominal muscles and prolong or shorten the duration of inspiration and exhalation, then his learning will be even more tortuous.

The above is my advice, but since no survey of Tai Chi would be complete without outlining the approach taken by some teachers, this chapter will look at their methods. My parting shot against such methods would be to refer to Yang Cheng-fu's advice to Cheng Man-ch'ing – relax, relax and then relax again – everything else will follow.

The role of the breath in the functioning of human beings has been documented for centuries in China, India, Japan and other countries. This documentation has always related to specific disciplines such as the cure of illness, training in Indian Yoga, the Taoist religion's search for immortality and so on. If a person is not ill, does not want to become an Indian Yogi or find immortality then it could be argued that the exercises described in books are not anything to do with him or her.

An inscription on a piece of jade from the Chou dynasty (1027–256 BC) speaks about holding the breath, the expansion of the breath, the solidification of the breath and the movement of the breath. Most of the references to breathing in subsequent writings relate it to the Tan T'ien, the spot just below the navel, in which it is said that Chi can be stored. The role of the breath in this storing of Chi was to assist the mind in bringing the Chi to this point. If the Chi could be so stored, then the theory is that this can lead to further psychic possibilities.

One of several modern researchers into breathing therapy is Tadashi Nakamura, a professor of clinical psychology of the Oriental Respiratory Research Institute. He attempted to correlate new theories, including primal scream therapy, with the older traditions of breathing therapy.

Nakamura began by showing the relationship between breathing and emotional states. When a person moves from a depressed to a happy frame of mind, the diaphragm movement increases and the lungs expand. In an experiment, it was suggested to some people with financial problems that they had found some large sums of money lying in the street. The diaphragm and lungs automatically responded as anticipated.

TAN T'IEN

As far as the exact location of the Tan T'ien is concerned, Tadashi Nakamura, a professor of clinical psychology of the Oriental Respiratory Research Institute, quotes various 'old books' and gives four different locations. One is 9cm below the navel, another between the kidneys and the navel itself, a third some 4cm below the navel and the fourth at the intersection of two acupuncture channels; one running round the waist and the other running down the front of the body. It is tempting to choose the last location because the Chinese character for T'ien, field, is like a rectangle with a vertical cross in it, and one feels that this crossing point could be related to the crossing of the two channels. Maybe in this case we should resist temptation and simply say that the Tan T'ien is near the navel and probably below it.

ENDOMORPHINS

Endorphin is a substance that calms down the organism and helps it to eliminate fear, as well as sensations of pain. One theory, which relates to the calming effects of deeper breathing over a prolonged period, suggests that deep breathing may produce greater amounts of endorphin than normal.

Further simple collation of existing data showed that lung function peaks in the majority of people around the age of 20 and that by the age of 60, it has reduced to the level of a nine-year-old. We can therefore appreciate that regular Tai Chi training, by inducing deep and relaxed breathing, may well counteract some of the effects of ageing. Without special athletic training or physical work, the quantity of air breathed in can be as little as 400cc, whereas with training, capacity can increase to 3,500cc.

The regulatory mechanism for breathing in the human nervous system is located in the medulla oblongata, near the occiput, where the skull meets the vertebrae of the spine. Good head-spine posture and good muscle tone of the region, as emphasized in both Tai Chi and the Alexander Technique, contribute to improved breathing. When Zen monks sit for long periods in meditation, the position of the head and spine plays an important role in the deep abdominal breathing that they follow. Tests showed that even though a Zen monk may breathe between only two and five times a minute, without strain, and a normal breathing rate may be say 18 times a minute, the number of litres of air inhaled and exhaled will be the same.

After a number of further experiments and comparison with the data of other workers in the field, Nakamura summarized the results of deeper breathing on the digestive organs, the circulation and the nervous system. In doing so, he confirmed the claims that have been made for some years by Tai Chi teachers, but in the more poetic language of the Chinese culture. Prolonged deeper breathing stimulates the stomach, liver, kidneys and intestines. A simple but welcome effect is to relieve constipation. It also assists in the absorption of nourishing substances by the digestive organs by affecting the capillary vessels, and promotes excretion by the kidneys. The circulation system is assisted by deep breathing because it helps prevent the accumulation of cholesterol and stimulates the activity of the red and white blood corpuscles. The absorption of oxygen and the elimination of carbon dioxide proceeds more efficiently.

The division of the nervous system into sympathetic and parasympathic, stimulation and sedation, is regulated by deep breathing and in this respect Nakamura cites the presence of Ki (the Japanese word for Chi). Ki, he maintains, is assisted in its work by better functioning of the respiratory system. At this point, Nakamura departs from his strict reliance on Western scientific methods and the use of statistical analysis and returns to the beliefs of his fathers.

Having laid down his proofs of the benefits of such breathing, Nakamura goes on to present a number of cautionary words about the use of breathing exercises. Here he makes a clear distinction between normal, healthy people and people who are unwell. Speaking of the latter, he says, 'Once under control [the breathing] they should endeavour to continue natural breathing.' Among the effects of deep

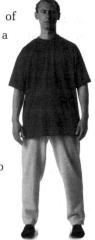

RIGHT DEEP RELAXED BREATHING STIMULATES THE VITAL ORGANS OF THE BODY.

BREATHING THERAPY

The ideal standing posture for breathing therapy is similar to that used by Kenichi Sawai of the Tai-ki-ken style of martial arts – feet apart, a little wider than the hips and the arms held in a horizontal 'circle' level with the shoulders. In this posture, a process is supposed to take place that is the same as the one found in the Chinese Tai Chi tradition. The Ki 'condenses' at the Tan T'ien, under the influence of the 'I' and the breath, and rises to the top of the head through the spine and also down to the tips of the toes.

The main idea in the beginning stage of this therapy is that during breathing one tries to bring the attention down to the Tan T'ien in order to feel free from thoughts in the brain. Nakamura quotes a saying that 'attention protects the Tanden' (Japanese for Tan T'ien). He explains a further benefit of focusing on the Tan T'ien by pointing out that it is near the solar plexus, a part of the nervous system whose tension is part of many undesirable emotional states.

breathing therapy, which can be adverse unless properly supervised, are dizziness and pain, variations in heart beat, temporary diminishing of the sense of taste, abnormal itching of the skin, wind, loosening of the bowels, nocturnal emissions and feelings of heaviness. People with arteriosclerosis and hypertension should be especially careful with breathing exercises.

Nakamura also touches on the use of visualization of the benefits expected from breathing therapy, a method used by holistic therapy centres. He likens this to bringing together the Ki and the 'I' (ee), the Chinese word for mind.

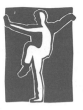

TAI CHI TODAY

CHAPTER ELEVEN

Since I first started Tai Chi, some time in 1968, the spread of the art throughout the world has been amazing. At that time there were few Westerners who had even heard of it, let alone seen it. As far as I know, there were only two people teaching the art in London and one of them was a visiting American. I leave aside the many Chinese who were possibly practising on their own and out of sight. Now most evening institutes have a Tai Chi class and many colleges have Tai Chi clubs.

The main style taught has been the Yang style, but in recent years the Chen style has become more popular, along with styles synthesized by the Chinese athletic organizations. Push Hands is becoming more widespread and Tai Chi Combat is getting a hold in various forms. Sadly, Pa-kua and Hsing-I have not shared in this rise in popularity. Many clubs insist that the students wear the traditional Chinese outfit for training, consisting of a jacket

LEFT SPECIAL CLOTHING IS NOT ESSENTIAL FOR TAI CHI. HOWEVER, STUDENTS SHOULD WEAR LOOSE, COMFORTABLE CLOTHING THAT ALLOWS COMPLETE FREEDOM OF MOVEMENT.

fastened by braid toggles and a Mandarin collar. Others allow casual clothes. The two most important points about clothing are the trousers and shoes. Trousers should allow freedom of movement, jeans are out, and shoes should give the foot a comfortable flat surface on which to rest so that there is no danger of over-balancing. Trainers with thick soles are a menace in this respect. They may be all right for jogging but not for Tai Chi.

I do not like the rubber or plastic soled Kung Fu shoe that is very popular with students. The impact on the ground is very dead and some of them are inclined to slip. I usually wear a pair of very old and comfortable leather shoes with a rubber sole.

Prices charged for Tai Chi lessons vary considerably. Evening institutes are the cheapest, but in private clubs one can pay much more. However, private teachers have overheads to meet that do not apply to institutions in the same way. It is also true to say that in many cases the standard of tuition in institutions is not always equal to that in private clubs, where the teacher is often full time and has a long background in martial arts. Many evening institutes have teachers who would not rate at all in martial arts circles. However, this is probably true in many other subjects as well as Tai Chi, and provided a teacher can do a form passably well, why not learn from him or her.

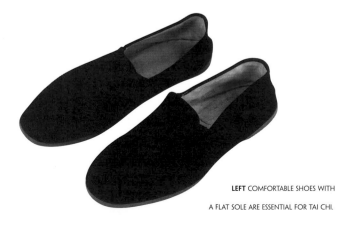

LEFT COMFORTABLE SHOES WITH
A FLAT SOLE ARE ESSENTIAL FOR TAI CHI.

In my experience, the fact that someone can do Tai Chi well does not mean that he is also a qualified historian, philosophy master, doctor, athletic coaching specialist or expert Taoist mystic. When you are in a pupil-teacher relationship with someone, your critical faculties may be blunted. If the teacher says something about Tai Chi that is perfectly accurate and true, then in the same sentence says something about medicine, history or philosophy, one might make some reservations about the second half.

As I hope this book has made clear, the world of Tai Chi today is like an enormous warehouse in which the past has accumulated. If a student wishes to understand it, he or she must start sorting it out for him or herself.

FURTHER READING

Chen Style Taiji Quan, compiled by Zhaohua Publishing House, Beijing, 1984

Chen, Yearning K, trans. Olson, Stuart Alve, *Tai Chi Sword, Sabre and Staff*, Bubbling Well Press, 1986

Cheng, Man-Jan, *Lao Tzu: My Words Are Very Easy To Understand*, North Atlantic Books, 1981

Chung-yan, Chang, *Creativity and Taoism*, Wildwood House, 1975

De Bary, William Theodore (compiler), *Sources of Chinese Tradition*, Vol 1, Columbia University Press, 1960

Ju-Pai, Dr Tseng, *Tai Chi Weapons*, Paul H Crompton Ltd, 1982

Kaptchuk, T, *Chinese Medicine: The Web That Has No Weaver*, Rider, 1983

Kushi, Michio, *The Book of Macrobiotics*, Japan Publications Inc., 1977

Man-Ching, Cheng, trans. Wile, Douglas, *Master Cheng's Thirteen Chapters on T'ai Chi Ch'uan*, Sweet Ch'i Press, 1982

Nakamura, Tadashi, *Oriental Breathing Therapy*, Japan Publications Inc., 1977

Needham, Joseph, *Science and Civilization in China*, Vol 2, Cambridge University Press, 1956

Sawai, Kenichi, *Taiki-Ken*, Japan Publications Inc., 1976

Shchutskii, I K, *Researches on the I-Ching*, Routledge, 1980

Smith, R W, *Chinese Boxing, Masters and Methods*, Kodansha, 1974

Stevens, John, *Abundant Peace*, Shambhala, 1987

Suzuki, D T, *Zen and Japanese Culture*, Princeton University Press, 1973

Ta-Kao, C H (translator), *Tao Te Ching*, Unwin, 1976

Veith, Ilsa (translator), *The Yellow Emperor's Book of Internal Medicine*, University of California Press, 1972

Wilhelm, Richard (translator), *I-Ching*, Routledge, 1965

Yu-Lan, Professor Fung, *A Short History of Chinese Philosophy*, Macmillan, 1948

GLOSSARY

Aikido A Japanese martial art employing body movements that in some instances resemble those of Push Hands of Tai Chi.

Blood A term used in traditional Chinese medicine to describe not only blood in the Western sense but also the various functions that it carries out.

Ch'an Buddhism A form of Buddhism peculiar to China, emphasizing direct experience of reality rather than thought, and based on a blending of Taoism and Buddhism.

Chen The name of the family that produced the Chen style of Tai Chi; more varied in speed, posture and combative application than any of the other styles.

Chi Vital energy, intrinsic energy, vitality that accompanies the activities of all life.

Chi Kung (Qi Gong) The art and science of cultivating the Chi in human beings.

Ching (Jing) A vital energy recognized by traditional Chinese medicine and directly related to the growth and development of human beings.

Five Animals An ancient form of Chi Kung using the imitated movements of animals, for example, tiger, deer, bear, monkey, crane, to promote health and longevity.

Five Elements Earth, fire, water, metal and wood, these represent five phases through which all processes are supposed to pass; a complex and at times controversial idea.

Fluids The most 'Yin' of all the substances in the human body recognized by Chinese traditional medicine. They include urine, sweat and saliva.

Form The sequences of unbroken movement used in Tai Chi to exercise the body, study the postures and cultivate the Chi.

Hsing I One of the three major internal martial arts of China. It uses an extensive range of animal movements and is the most vigorous of the three.

I-Ching An ancient book of divination, with extensive commentaries and interpretations, which has greatly influenced Chinese culture.

Nei Chia An expression meaning 'internal school' (of martial arts) that has sometimes been used, probably erroneously, to describe Tai Chi.

Pakua (Bagna) An expression meaning 'eight trigrams'. In martial arts it refers to a form of combat and training supposedly based on the symbols found in the *I-Ching*. One of the three major internal martial arts of China.

Posture A misleading term suggesting a static pose in the Tai Chi Forms. In reality the 'postures' are simply distinct movements found in a Form.

Push Hands A two person exercise used in Tai Chi training to develop a sense of the interplay of yin and yang, yielding and pushing.

Shen The finest energy in human beings according to traditional Chinese medicine. It has been translated as 'spirit'.

Sun A style of Tai Chi invented by Sun Lu-T'ang; now almost extinct.

Taiki-Ken The Japanese rendering of Tai Chi Chuan and also the name of a style of combat taught in Japan based on the internal martial arts of China.

Taoism A form of Chinese philosophy and self-cultivation.

Tao te Ching A book of Taoist wisdom, popularly attributed to the sage Lao-tzu, but more likely a compilation of writings from various sources.

Trigram An arrangement of three parallel broken or unbroken lines denoting yin or yang energy, combined in pairs to form the hexagrams (six lines) of the *I-Ching*.

Wu The name of the family that produced the Wu style of Tai Chi.

Wushu An expression meaning 'martial arts' and generally preferred by purists to the better known Western usage of the word Kung Fu.

Yang The name of the family that produced the Yang style of Tai Chi, which is today the best known outside China.

Yin-Yang A fundamental division of forces into opposites: female-male, dark-light, yielding-aggressive. The name of a school of Chinese philosophy.

Zen-Ch'an Buddhism This was introduced to Japan over a period of time, it took root and was developed along Japanese lines and is known as Zen Buddhism.

Useful Addresses

EUROPE
Taijiquan and
Qigong Federation
for Europe
Web:www.taijiquan-
qigung.com

UK
Paul Crompton
94 Felsham Road
London
SW15 1DQ

Patrick Harries
21 Grosvenor Road
Stalbridge
Dorset
DT10 2PL

Ronnie Robinson
69 Kilpatrick
Gardens
Clarkston
Glasgow
G76 7RF
Tel: +44(0) 1647
231477

Mike Tabrett
6 Swanns Terrace
Cambridge
CB1 3LX

FRANCE
Féderation Française
des Tai Chi
Chuan Traditionnels
78 Rue Saint Honoré
75001 Paris
Tel: 01 45 43 03 96

THE NETHERLANDS
Pierre de Cat
Postbus 2271800
AE Alcmaar
Email:mailiing@taiji
quanqigong.com

Strichting Taijiquan
Nederland
Postbus 13 26 4,
3507 LG
Utrecht
Tel: 030 289 6336
Publishers of
Nieuwsbrief
magazine.

US
Universal Tai Chi
Chuan Association
Contact: Ben Lo
2901 Clement Street
San Francisco
CA 94121

William Chen
2 Washington
Square Village
#10J, New York
NY 10012
Tel: (212) 675 2816

Yang's Martial Arts
Association
Contact: Dr Yang
Jwing Ming
28 Hyde Park
Avenue
Jamaica Plain
MA 02130-4132
Tel: (1-617) 524
8892

INDEX

125

LOOK AT LIFE...
with a NEW PERSPECTIVE

A series of comprehensive introductions
to key mind, body, spirit subjects

★ **STYLISH AND ACCESSIBLE** ★

★ **STRAIGHTFORWARD AND PRACTICAL** ★

★ **CONTEMPORARY TWO COLOUR DESIGN WITH ILLUSTRATIONS** ★

BOOKS AVAILABLE IN THE SERIES:

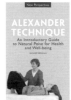

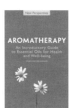

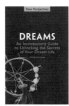

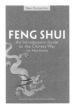

| 86204 629 8 | 86204 630 1 | 86204 667 0 | 86204 628 X

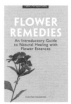

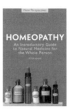

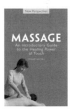

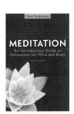

| 86204 664 6 | 86204 663 8 | 86204 626 3 | 86204 627 1

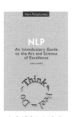

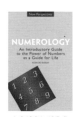

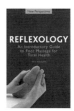

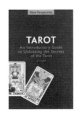

| 86204 668 9 | 86204 625 5 | 86204 665 4 | 86204 673 5

ALSO AVAILABLE IN THIS SERIES: **ASTROLOGY** 1 86204 666 2, **BUDDHISM** 1 86204 764 2, **CHAKRAS** 1 86204 765 0,
COLOUR THERAPY 1 86204 766 9, **CRYSTAL THERAPY** 1 86204 739 1, **HERBAL REMEDIES** 1 86204 767 7,
I CHING 1 86204 763 4, **NUTRITIONAL THERAPY** 1 86204 740 5, **RUNES** 1 86204 762 6,
SHAMANISM 1 86204 761 8, **TAI CHI** 1 86204 760 X, **YOGA** 1 86204 759 6.